Common Contact Lens Complications:

Their Recognition and Management

Common Contact Lens Complications:

Their Recognition and Management

Lyndon W. Jones PhD FCOptom DCLP DOrth FIACLE FAAO

Associate Professor
School of Optometry, University of Waterloo, Ontario, Canada
Associate Director
Centre for Contact Lens Research, University of Waterloo, Ontario, Canada

Deborah A. Jones BSc FCOptom DCLP FAAO

Lecturer
School of Optometry, University of Waterloo, Ontario, Canada
Research Optometrist
Centre for Contact Lens Research, University of Waterloo, Ontario, Canada

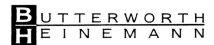

OXFORD   AUCKLAND   BOSTON   JOHANNESBURG   MELBOURNE   NEW DELHI

Butterworth-Heinemann
Linacre House, Jordan Hill, Oxford OX2 8DP
225 Wildwood Avenue, Woburn, MA 01801-2041
A division of Reed Educational and Professional Publishing Ltd

℞ A member of the Reed Elsevier plc group

First published 2000

© Reed Educational and Professional Publishing Ltd 2000

British Library Cataloguing in Publication Data
Jones, Lyndon
 Common contact lens complications: their recognition and
 management
 1. Contact lenses – Complications
 I. Title   II. Jones, Deborah
 617.7'523

Library of Congress Cataloguing in Publication Data
Jones, Lyndon
 Common contact lens complications: their recognition and management/Lyndon
 Jones, Deborah Jones
 p. cm
 Includes bibliographical references and index.
 ISBN 0 7506 3542 8
 1. Contact lenses – Complications.   I. Jones, Deborah, lecturer.   II. Title.
 [DNLM: 1. Contact Lenses – adverse effects.   2. Eye Diseases – complications.   3. Eye
 Diseases – therapy.   4. Eye Injuries – therapy.   WW 355 J77c 2000]
 RE977.C6 J62
 617.7'523 – dc21   99-044549

ISBN 0 7506 3542 8
Data manipulation by David Gregson Associates, Beccles, Suffolk
Printed and bound in Italy

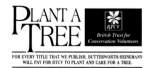

Contents

Introduction

It is estimated that approximately 80 million people world-wide wear contact lenses. Whilst the vast majority of patients wear lenses without complications, others manifest problems, many of which are subtle in nature. If clinicians induce complications then it is their duty to recognize the problem and institute appropriate management strategies to alleviate the condition. Such action will frequently prevent the problem becoming worse and should allow the patient to continue wearing lenses in a problem-free manner.

The principal aim of this book is to provide a handy reference guide to the recognition and management of contact lens complications that are commonly seen in everyday clinical practice. Its production was driven by our awareness of the need for a simple pocket-guide to the management of contact lens related complications. Some of the complications may not be directly attributable to contact lenses, but their presence will in some way have an impact on either contact lens fitting or their successful wear.

The book consists of two distinct sections. The first examines the slit lamp biomicroscope and describes how it may be best utilized to recognize subtle corneal and conjunctival anomalies. The second describes a variety of commonly seen complications, broadly outlines their aetiology and clearly defines a list of management strategies. It is not intended to provide a fully referenced guide to the aetiology of contact lens complications but rather a guide which practitioners and students can have readily at hand in the consulting room. For further details readers are referred to a list of key references at the end of each complication.

These references are deliberately limited to a minimal number and are considered to be the references that would quickly expand the clinician's knowledge in the area and, as such, are frequently review articles or book chapters.

Many people have personally helped us over the years with our understanding of both the recognition and management of contact lens complications. Notable amongst these have been three people who were initially mentors, subsequently colleagues and now considered good friends – Keith Edwards, Ian Davies and Nathan Efron. These people were all instrumental in exciting our interest in contact lenses and helping us during our formative years to understand the need to be critical of our approach in the management of contact lens patients.

Finally we would like to thank the long list of people who contributed their photographs so willingly to this book. A picture really does say a thousand words and good photographs of contact lens complications are an essential item in a book of this type.

Lyndon and Deborah Jones

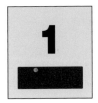

The slit lamp biomicroscope: principles and techniques

The slit lamp biomicroscope is the most important instrument in contact lens practice, playing an essential role in the preliminary assessment and aftercare of the prospective and existing contact lens wearer. The opportunities for using the slit lamp within the routine eye examination are also numerous and diverse. With the appropriate use of supplementary lenses and/or viewing techniques the instrument may be used to assess the condition of the vitreous, lens and retina from posterior pole to the ora serrata. Various ancillary instruments will permit examination of the anterior chamber angle, measurement of intra-ocular pressure, and assessment of corneal sensitivity and thickness.

This chapter will review the biomicroscope and the principal techniques used for ocular examination. Particular attention will be paid to the illumination techniques necessary to recognize conditions frequently seen in contact lens wearers and the methods available for recording such observations.

The instrument

The instrument consists of a separate illumination system (the slit lamp) and viewing system (the biomicroscope) which have a common focal point and centre of rotation. A height control moves both systems simultaneously and focusing and lateral movements are achieved via a joystick. This common control feature facilitates rapid and accurate positioning of the slit beam on the area of interest and ensures that the microscope and illumination system are simultaneously in focus.

Illumination system

Virtually all slit lamp manufacturers have adopted the Koeller illumination system, which is optically almost identical to that of a 35 mm slide projector.[1]

- A bright illumination system (producing approximately 600 000 lux) is a fundamental requirement for a slit lamp if subtle conditions are to be clearly seen. While halogen or xenon lamps are more expensive than tungsten lamps, they are the preferred illumination source as they provide a brighter light, last longer, have better colour rendering and generate less heat. Illumination brightness is controlled by a rheostat or multi-position switch such that brightness can be adjusted to obtain the correct balance between patient comfort and optimal visibility of the area of interest.

- The slit within the illumination system must have sharply demarcated edges and be adjustable in a variety of ways:

  1. The slit width and height must be easily adjustable such that any shaped patch from a slit to a circle may be projected, as this will increase the variety of illumination methods possible. A graduated slit width is particularly useful when measuring the size of a lesion.

  2. An ability to rotate the lamp housing such that the slit may be used in meridians away from the vertical is useful, particularly if a protractor scale is included. Such a system enables, for example, the angle of rotation of a soft toric lens away from the vertical to be accurately measured.

  3. The slit beam must have the facility to be displaced or offset sideways ('decoupled'). This ability to break the

linkage between the illumination and observation systems facilitates indirect illumination techniques.

● A number of filters are incorporated into the illumination system and are used to enhance the visibility of certain conditions:

1. Green ('red-free') filter – this is used to enhance contrast when looking for corneal and iris vascularization, since red vessels appear black if viewed through such a filter. In addition, it may be used to increase the visibility of rose bengal staining on both the cornea and conjunctiva.

2. Neutral density (ND) filters – these are used to reduce the beam brightness and increase comfort for the patient.

3. Polarizing filters – these reduce unwanted specular reflections and can be useful to enhance the visibility of subtle defects.

4. Diffusing filter – this diffuses the illumination source over a wide area and is used to provide broad, unfocused illumination for low magnification viewing of the general ocular surface.

5. Cobalt blue filter – this filter's main use is to provide a suitable means of exciting sodium fluorescein for examination of ocular surface integrity. Illumination of fluorescein with cobalt blue light of 460–490 nm produces a greenish light of maximum emission 520 nm. Any abraded area will absorb fluorescein and display a fluorescent green area against a general blue background (Figure 1.1). The filter is occasionally used on its own to aid in the diagnosis of keratoconus. A frequent finding in this corneal ectasia is Fleischer's ring, which is formed by an annular iron deposition within the stroma at the base of the cone. The iron pigment is often difficult to see in white light but will usually appear in greater contrast when viewed through the cobalt blue filter.

6. Kodak Wratten No. 12 (yellow) filter – this is not a

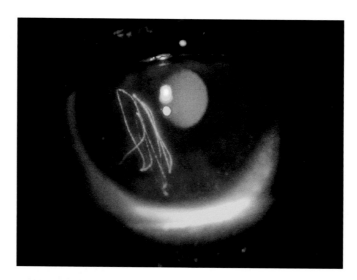

Figure 1.1   Corneal staining from a foreign body trapped under a rigid lens. The abraded areas are clearly seen through the uptake of fluorescein.

filter contained within the illumination system but a barrier filter placed in front of the viewing system. It significantly enhances the contrast of any fluorescent staining observed with the cobalt blue filter as it allows transmission of the green fluorescent light but blocks the blue light reflected from the corneal surface.[2,3] Custom-made barrier filters for certain slit lamps are available from the manufacturers (Figure 1.2). Inexpensive hand-held versions may be constructed by using a cardboard mask and Lee filters No. 101 (yellow), which can be purchased from a variety of suppliers, including those shown in Table 1.1.

Table 1.1   Sources of yellow filters

Company	Address	Telephone	Fax
Lee Filters UK	Central Way, Walworth Industrial Estate, Andover Hants SP10 5AN, UK	01264 366245	01264 355058
Lee Filters USA	2237 North Hollywood Way, Burbank, CA 91505, USA	818 238 1220	818 238 1228
John Barry Group Pty Ltd	1 McLachlan Way, Artarmon, NSW 2064, Australia	612 9439 6955	612 9439 2375

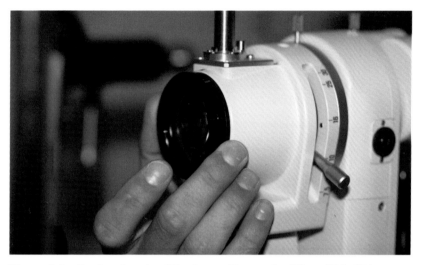

Figure 1.2   Custom barrier filter in position on the Nikon FS3 slit lamp. The slider for the zoom magnification system is also clearly seen.

The microscope

The second prerequisite for a slit lamp is a viewing system that provides a clear image of the eye and has sufficient magnification for the practitioner to view all structures of interest. Magnification is an important issue and the slit lamp should be capable of providing magnifications of up to 40×, which may be achieved through interchangeable eyepieces and/or variable magnification of the slit lamp objective.[1] Magnification greater than this level is usually unnecessary and is often counter-productive, as small involuntary eye movements will render the image too unstable to view. Ideally the practitioner should be able to change magnification swiftly and easily, which gives slit lamps with three or more objectives an advantage. Zoom systems have the added advantage of allowing the practitioner to focus on a particular structure without losing sight of it during changes in magnification.

It is important to remember that the magnified image must also be clear and the importance of choosing a slit lamp with a high quality optical system cannot be over-stressed. Ideally the microscope should have excellent resolution and a good depth of field. However, these factors are inversely linked and so a compromise must be accepted. The resolution of the image is the most important factor and is governed by the numerical aperture (NA) of the microscope, which is dependent upon:[4]

- The diameter of the objective – the bigger the better, but bigger diameters result in peripheral aberrations.

- The working distance – the shorter the better, but shorter working distances result in problems with supplementary lenses and equipment that need to be interposed between the microscope and the patient's eye.

- The refractive index of the medium between the objective lenses and the eye – the higher the better, but it is impractical to place a high refractive index fluid between the microscope and the patient.

- The wavelength of light – the shorter the better, but this will influence the colour rendering properties of the eye.

Illumination and observation techniques

Mastering the available illumination techniques possible with the slit lamp is essential if the instrument is to be used to its full potential, and practice with the instrument is critical to becoming comfortable with its subtle but extensive variety of uses. In reality it is impractical to completely dissociate the viewing techniques, as in one field of view several different methods of illumination simultaneously present themselves. The experienced observer is then able to assimilate useful information without having to necessarily resort to different physical adjustments of the slit lamp. It is important to remember that the optical effects produced by the incident beam of light depend upon the tissues illuminated and their transparency, as reflection, scattering or absorption can all occur to various degrees.

This section will briefly describe the ideal set-up for each of the three principal illumination methods.

Diffuse illumination

A ground-glass filter is placed in the focused light beam of the slit lamp. This defocuses and diffuses the light to give a broad, even illumination over the entire field of view and is generally used to provide low magnification views of the anterior segment (Figures 1.3 and 1.4). Typical uses include viewing soft contact lens fitting characteristics, contact lens deposits, external eyelid anomalies and general conjunctival appearance.

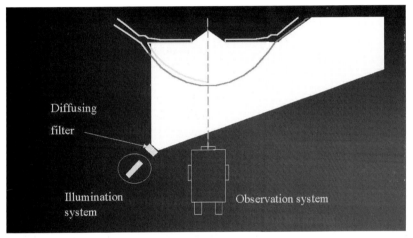

Figure 1.3   Diagrammatic representation of diffuse illumination.

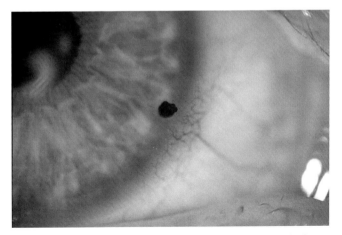

Figure 1.4   Diffuse illumination view of an embedded metallic foreign body in the cornea. Note how the depth of the foreign body cannot be determined using this technique.

Direct focal illumination

This describes any illumination technique where the slit beam and viewing system are focused coincidentally. The illumination beam is turned up as brightly as possible (ensuring that the patient remains comfortable) and placed at a separation of 40–60° on the side of the microscope corresponding to the section of the cornea to be viewed. The beam is swept smoothly across the ocular surface and the illumination system moved across to the opposite side as the beam crosses the mid-point of the cornea. Typically a beam width of 2–3 mm is chosen initially and this is reduced as an area of interest is discovered. Whilst scanning the external surface, a low to medium magnification is initially chosen and the magnification increased if any areas of interest are noted.

Parallelepiped

Using the set-up described above, an illuminating beam of 0.5–2.0 mm in width is scanned over the ocular surface (Figure 1.5). This permits assessment of the location, width and height of any object within the cornea or adjacent structures (Figure 1.6). This is the most commonly used direct illumination technique and is employed to assess, for example, corneal scarring, infiltrates and corneal staining.

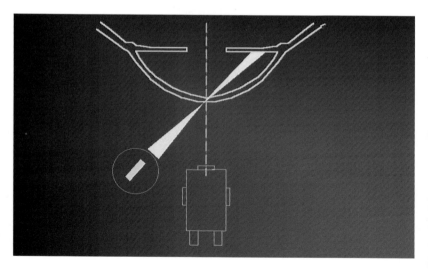

Figure 1.5   Diagrammatic representation of a parallelepiped.

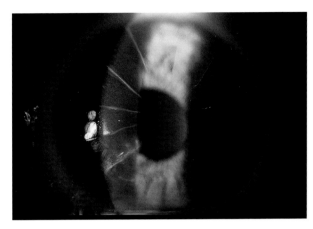

Figure 1.6 Wide parallelepiped view of radial keratotomy scars. Note how it is not possible to judge the depth of the incisions with this technique. Also note how the scars are not visible to the right of the direct beam in the light reflected from the iris. (Picture courtesy of Rosaline Robinson.)

Optic section

Once an area or object of interest is located the beam width is narrowed to approximately 0.2 mm to 'cross-section' the corneal tissue. This provides the ability to accurately assess the depth of an object within the corneal layers (Figure 1.7). Typical uses include assessment of the depth of a foreign body, location of a corneal scar (Figure 1.8) and determining whether tissue within an area of staining is excavated, flat or raised.

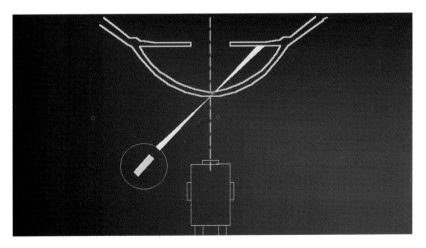

Figure 1.7 Diagrammatic representation of an optic section.

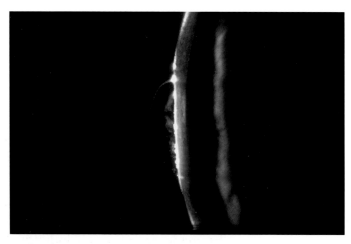

Figure 1.8   Optic section of a corneal scar. Note how the use of this technique clearly enables the location of the scar to be noted and how the cornea is thinned centrally. (Picture courtesy of Desmond Fonn.)

Oblique illumination

This is infrequently used in contact lens practice, but is nonetheless a useful technique. This illumination method is achieved by setting up a parallelepiped and then moving the illumination system away from the observation system until the angle between them is close to 90°. The illumination arm is adjusted until the light beam is almost tangential to the object of interest. Any raised areas cast a shadow and this technique is particularly useful for viewing subtle defects within the iris architecture and subtle epithelial changes.

Conical beam

This technique is principally used to assess the presence or absence of inflammatory cells and protein ('flare') in the anterior chamber as a result of anterior uveitis. A narrow parallelepiped of approximately 1 mm in width is set up, the height of the beam is reduced to 1–2 mm by interposing an aperture within the illumination system and all room illumination is extinguished. The anterior chamber is scanned at low to medium magnification by systematically changing focus from the anterior lens surface to the cornea. Any inflammatory cells appear as white/yellow particles within the anterior chamber.[5]

Specular reflection

This is a specific case of a parallelepiped set-up, where the angle of the incident slit beam is equal to the angle of the observation axis through one of the oculars. At this angle (typically 40–50°) the illumination beam is reflected from the smooth surfaces of the anterior segment and provides a mirror-like reflection (Figure 1.9). These images occur at every interface between structures of different refractive indices. It is typically used to view the endothelium (Figure 1.10), tear film quality, the 'orange-peel' appearance of the anterior lens surface and front surface wetting of a contact lens. It is important to realize that even at ×40 magnification only a gross clinical judgement of the endothelium can be made as, although individual cells can be seen, they are very small.

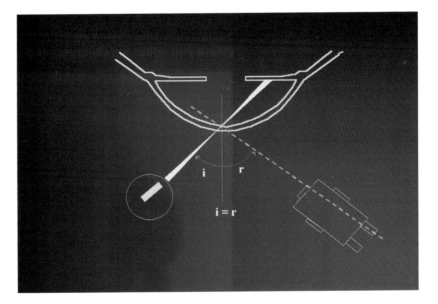

Figure 1.9   Diagrammatic representation of specular reflection.

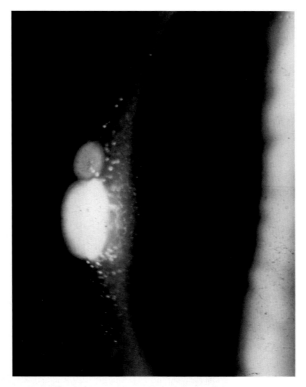

Figure 1.10 Specular reflection view of endothelial guttata, which are clearly visible to the right of the specular reflex.

Indirect illumination

This refers to any technique where the focus of the illuminating beam does not coincide with the focal point of the observation system. This can be achieved by 'uncoupling' the instrument and manually displacing the slit beam to the side. However, most experienced observers will set up a direct illumination of the section adjacent to that of interest and view to the side of the directly illuminated area.

Several specific illuminations are available, as outlined below.

Sclerotic scatter

This technique is used to investigate any subtle changes in corneal clarity occurring over a large area, such as central corneal oedema. The slit lamp is set up for a wide-angle parallelepiped (45–60°) and the viewing system focused centrally. The beam is manually offset ('decoupled') and focused on the limbus. The slit beam is totally internally reflected across the cornea and a bright limbal glow is seen around the entire cornea (Figure 1.11). Any specific area of abnormality such as a corneal scar will interrupt the beam in its passage and produce a light reflection in the otherwise dark cornea (Figure 1.12).

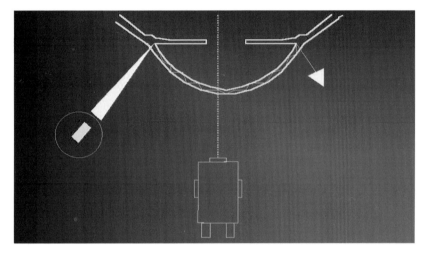

Figure 1.11   Diagrammatic representation of sclerotic scatter.

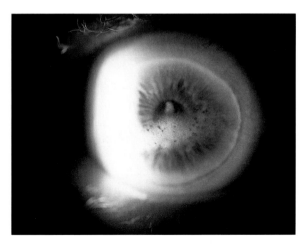

Figure 1.12   Band keratopathy made visible by the use of sclerotic scatter. The area over which the keratopathy extends is clearly seen using this technique.

Retro illumination

This refers to any technique in which light is reflected from the iris, anterior lens surface or retina and is used to back-illuminate an area more anteriorly positioned. The area may be seen against a light background (direct retro; Figure 1.13) or a dark background (indirect retro; Figure 1.14), depending on whether the illumination and viewing systems are coincident or not. The commonest type is direct retro, in which corneal opacities will appear black against a bright field. This technique is particularly useful for examining epithelial microcysts, neovascularization, scars, degenerations and dystrophies (Figure 1.15).

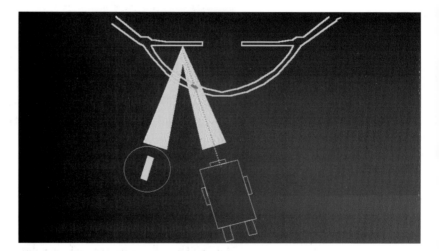

Figure 1.13 Diagrammatic representation of direct retro illumination.

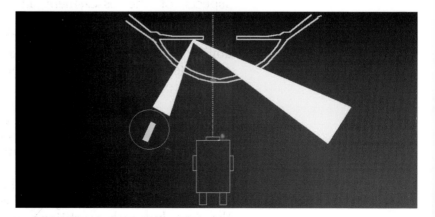

Figure 1.14 Diagrammatic representation of indirect retro illumination.

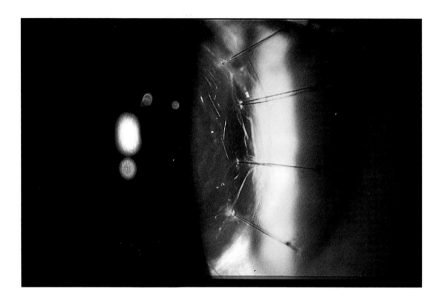

Figure 1.15 Slit lamp view of sutures in a patient following penetrating keratoplasty. Note how the sutures and corneal wrinkling are seen in indirect illumination from light reflected from the iris.

The slit lamp routine

As with all aspects of ocular examination, practitioners should develop a routine that enables them to cover all aspects of the assessment in a logical, systematic and consistent manner. The slit lamp examination of the eye requires several different illumination techniques, and the ability to detect and diagnose anterior segment conditions often depends upon the skill of the observer to use the correct technique. The order of the examination will vary from one practitioner to another. Usually, the examination will start with low magnification and diffuse illumination for general observation, with the magnification increasing and more specific illumination techniques being employed to view structures in more detail.

The typical routine detailed below is suggested as one that should flow smoothly from one group of structures to the next, but each practitioner will inevitably develop their own variation.

Overall view: low magnification, wide diffuse beam

The examination should begin with a number of sweeps across the anterior segment and adnexa, whilst using a broad diffused beam and low magnification. The lid margins and lashes should be examined for signs of marginal blepharitis or hordeolum and the patency of the meibomium glands assessed by gently squeezing the lids. The bulbar conjunctiva is then assessed for hyperaemia and the presence of any abnormality such as pinguecula or pterygium. Finally, the superior and inferior palpebral conjunctiva are examined to check for hyperaemia, follicles and papillae.

Cornea and limbal examination: medium magnification, 2 mm wide beam

The diffusing filter is removed and the corneal examination begins with a sclerotic scatter to examine the cornea for gross opacification. The illumination and viewing systems are then recoupled and a series of sweeps carried out across the cornea. The limbus is examined by observing the limbal vasculature to assess the degree of physiological corneal vascularization (blood vessels overlaying clear cornea) and differentiating this from neovascularization (new blood vessels growing into clear cornea). Blood vessels are seen in both direct illumination and indirect retro illumination, looking to the side of the illuminated area of the cornea. Once the limbus has been assessed the cornea is examined with a parallelepiped to look for any gross abnormalities before narrowing the beam and increasing the magnification to examine the cornea in greater detail.

Corneal examination: high magnification, narrow beam

An optic section is obtained and, with high magnification, the slit lamp is systematically swept from side to side across the cornea to look for features of particular interest. At this point a number of illumination techniques will simultaneously be used. In addition to direct illumination to look for any subtle opacification, stromal striae and folds in Descemet's membrane, retro illumination will be used to look for the presence of microcysts, and the endothelium and tear film will be observed by specular reflection.

Staining examination

It is essential that the cornea be examined with various stains during contact lens aftercare checks[6] and in cases where patients complain of dry eyes; no contact lens aftercare should be considered complete without a staining examination taking place. Sodium fluorescein is a vital stain which stains damaged epithelial tissue and is the best means of judging corneal integrity. Rose bengal is an iodine derivative of fluorescein which binds to mucus and cellular components. It is useful in the diagnosis of dry eye, in which it is seen binding to degenerate cells on the corneal surface. Lissamine green is a relatively new vital stain which has a similar action to rose bengal but does not sting on installation.

Further information on slit lamp technique may be obtained from Morris and Stone,[7–9] Chauhan[4] and Veys and Davies.[10]

Recording of clinical observations

Of equal importance to carrying out the examination is the recording of the results obtained. In law, if an action is not recorded it is not deemed to have taken place, and practitioners must attempt to record and quantify what observations have been made. It is vitally important to ensure that such measurements are reproducible and repeatable if they are to be used successfully. Practitioners constantly record slit lamp observations in order to make clinical decisions. Recording findings using descriptive terms such as 'acceptable', 'slight', 'bumpy' or 'smooth' are too subjective in nature and are likely to result in variations both over time and between practitioners. A suitable system or systems must be used if the change in such clinical observations is to be accurately monitored.

One option is to physically measure the size of the object of interest. For example, blood vessel infiltration into the

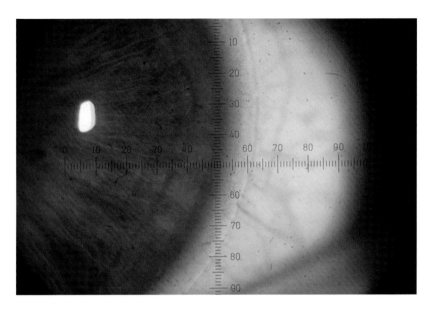

Figure 1.16   Use of a graticule eye-piece to measure soft contact lens movement and diameter.

cornea can be directly recorded by using a graduated graticule placed within the objective eyepiece. Some slit lamp manufacturers produce custom-made graticule eyepieces, but these are often expensive. An alternative suggestion involves converting the spare eyepieces often provided with slit lamps into dedicated graticule eyepieces, which are subsequently used when a measurement is required (Figure 1.16). These spare eyepieces can be converted relatively inexpensively by obtaining graticules from a variety of sources, including those listed in Table 1.2.

Certain objects may be simply counted. For example, the progression of stromal striae or epithelial microcysts may

Table 1.2   Sources of eyepiece graticules

Company	Address	Telephone	Fax.	E-mail
Pyser (SGI) Ltd (Graticulus Division)	Fircroft Way, Edenbridge, Kent TN8 6HA, UK	01732 864863	01732 865544	–
EMS	PO Box 251, 321 Morris Road, Fort Washington, PA 19034, USA	215 646 1566	215 646 8931	sgkcck@aol.com

be monitored by physically counting them. However, the majority of slit lamp observations can be neither counted nor measured. The most reliable recording technique for use with features that cannot be measured depends upon the practitioner assigning grading scales to their clinical observations.[11] Each observation may be regarded as part of a continuous scale, which is assigned a grade based on the clinical observation. This grade serves as a standard by which any future observation can be judged.

One of the most well described options is to use a continuous five-point scale[11], such as that shown in Table 1.3.

Table 1.3 Example of a five-point scale for grading observations

Numerical	Descriptive	Meaning
Grade 0	Normal	No action
Grade 1	Slight	Not clinically significant
Grade 2	Moderate	May require intervention
Grade 3	Severe	Requires intervention
Grade 4	Very severe	Requires medical intervention

More sensitive results are found if the scale is expanded to cover a range from 0 to 10.[12,13] One possible adaptation of the scale described in Table 1.3 is to use plus or minus increments (e.g. 0, 1−, 1, 1+),[13] which would change the scale from a five-point scale to a nine-point scale. This scale may be modified to include all the major clinical findings observed during a slit lamp examination. Several grading systems have been published,[14–16] but practitioners can easily devise their own. Recently the subject of grading has received considerable interest due to the release of grading systems based on diagrams[17] or photographs (from the Cornea and Contact Lens Research Unit, Sydney, Australia). The use of picture scales (particularly when used with a decimalized scoring system) reduces inter- and intra-observer variability,[18] offers better repeatability than verbal scales[19] and is now considered the preferred method of grading slit lamp observations in the absence of photographic means.

Additional techniques

In addition to examining the anterior corneal surface the slit lamp is an extremely flexible instrument and may be used for many other purposes. Complete coverage of the variety of uses for the slit lamp is outside the realm of this review, but the principal areas are worthy of mention.

Intra-ocular pressure

Applanation tonometry remains the 'gold standard' to which other, newer forms of tonometry are compared. Attachment of an applanation tonometer enables the practitioner to accurately assess intra-ocular pressures.[20]

Pachometry

The pachometer attachment is useful in assessing corneal oedema in contact lens wear, corneal thickness prior to refractive surgery and in keratoconic patients to monitor the progression of the corneal thinning. It is based on the measurement of the apparent thickness of the optical section, and its popularity is largely based on the commercial availability of a pachometer attachment for the Haag–Streit slit lamp. Two modifications to the pachometer to improve its accuracy include the use of two small light sources to ensure that the incident beam is normal to the corneal surface[21] and an electronic transducer to take a direct measurement from the optical scale.[22]

Anterior chamber depth estimation

A fuller review of this topic is given by Barrett and McGraw.[23]

van Herrick's technique

This is used to provide an indirect assessment of the anterior chamber (AC) angle.[24] It requires no specific instrumentation but is a very useful slit lamp technique to master, particularly in hypermetropic patients in which the angle appears shallow. It makes the assumption that there is a relationship between the AC depth and width, in which 'deep' ACs have a wide angle. A narrow corneal section is produced at the limbus and the width of the corneal section is used as the unit for estimating the AC angle width. If the width between the endothelium and iris surface is equal to or greater than the corneal section width then the angle is assumed to be wide open (grade 4). If the width is less than a quarter of the corneal section width then the angle is dangerously narrow (grade 1) and necessitates further examination.

Slit lamp method

This technique was developed by Smith[25] and is explained in full by Barrett and McGraw.[23] The biomicroscope is placed directly ahead of the patient and the illumination system is located 60° to the temporal side of the patient. A 1–2 mm wide slit beam is orientated horizontally and focused on the cornea, with a second image of the slit being simultaneously seen on the anterior lens capsule/iris. The slit length is slowly increased until the two slits just touch. The slit length which yields just touching images is converted to an anterior chamber depth by multiplying the value by a constant of 1.4.

Gonioscopy

This is the technique used to directly examine the anterior chamber.[26–29] It is important in the diagnosis of closed-angle glaucoma and in certain iris pathologies. The equipment consists of a contact device that has a mirror to direct light from the illumination system into the anterior chamber angle and is rotated to view the entire angle. A direct estimation of the anterior chamber angle is possible, but the technique necessitates application of a local anaesthetic and requires practice to become proficient at its use.

Examination of the crystalline lens

Early changes to the lens are easily detected with the slit lamp using a parallelepiped, particularly following dilation. Nuclear sclerotic changes are distinguished by a 'yellowy-green' reflex and cortical and posterior subcapsular changes may be easily differentiated.[30] Slit lamp examination is also useful in the detection of posterior capsular opacification following extracapsular extraction and implantation. This may require subsequent YAG laser capsulotomy to clear the opacified capsular material.

Examination of the vitreous

Following dilation, the slit lamp can prove invaluable in detecting changes to the vitreous. Patients presenting with complaints of sudden photopsia and floaters should be examined for the presence of 'tobacco dust' in the anterior vitreous.[31,32] These are pigment cells and are strongly suggestive of a retinal tear. An annular opacity (Weiss' ring) represents a ring of glial tissue detached from the margin of the optic disc and is pathognomonic of posterior vitreous detachment. Such findings require a mandatory and thorough examination of the posterior peripheral fundus to rule out the possibility of retinal tears.[33,34]

Fundus examination

Non-contact

Bi-aspheric positive power lenses are used to convert the slit lamp into a binocular indirect ophthalmoscope and are particularly useful for obtaining a high power binocular view of the optic disc and macula. The condensing lens powers most commonly used are +60D, +78D and +90D. The primary magnification is highest for the +60D lens (approximately ×1) and fields of view of up to 120° are possible with specially developed lens types. The slit lamp allows variable magnification of the image, which is higher than that provided by a conventional indirect ophthalmoscope.[35-37] Other less frequently used methods include the myopic Hruby lens (−55D) and the positive El Bayadi lens (+55D).[38,39]

Contact

Mirrored lenses are used in conjunction with the slit lamp to view the fundus, and are typically employed to view structures in the far periphery that are not visible with the direct ophthalmoscope.[38,40,41] The classical Goldmann three-mirror lens is a contact device with three mirrors that are progressively used to examine the posterior fundus. Its major disadvantage over the non-contact technique is the requirement for corneal anaesthesia prior to use, which makes it an inconvenient procedure for rapid and/or routine assessment.

Photography and video recording

Photography of the eye provides an extremely accurate means of recording findings. A 35 mm camera can either be incorporated into the slit lamp itself or attached as an add-on. Conventional slit lamps can easily be converted by attaching the camera in place of one of the eyepieces of the microscope system. An alternative to still photography is to add a video attachment. The decreasing size of video cameras makes this a highly practical option. In addition to providing an instant picture, which may be of value to demonstrate specific points to the patient, the camera/video may also be adapted to aid measurement for research purposes. The newest development within this field is that of digital imaging. This technology uses a video camera or digital camera to obtain an image which is then stored on a computer. This technique has significant advantages in that the image is obtained immediately, image storage and retrieval is far simpler than with photographs or video-segments and comparisons from one visit to the next are easily obtained.

Further information on photography,[42–47] videography[48] and imaging[49–51] can be obtained from the references.

Acknowledgements

The author would like to acknowledge Jane Veys, Philippe Betran and Ian Davies for their invaluable assistance in compiling this chapter, in particular with the production of the line diagrams. Figures 1.3, 1.5, 1.7, 1.9, 1.11, 1.13 and 1.14 are adapted from Zantos and Cox.[16]

References

1. Henson, D. (1996). Slit lamps. In *Optometric Instrumentation*, Vol. 1 (ed. Henson, D.), pp. 138–161. Butterworth-Heinemann, London.
2. Courtney, R. and Lee, J. (1982). Predicting ocular intolerance of a contact lens solution by use of a filter system enhancing fluorescein staining detection. *ICLC*, **9**(5), 302–310.
3. Back, A. (1988). Corneal staining with contact lens wear. *J Brit Contact Lens Assoc Trans Ann Clin Conf*, pp. 16–18.
4. Chauhan, K. (1999). The slit lamp. *Optician*, **217**(5692), 24–30.
5. Cullom, R. and Chang, B. (1994). Vitreous examination for cells. In *The Wills Eye Manual*, Vol. 1 (eds Cullom, R. and Chang, B.), p. 458. JB Lippincott, Philadelphia.
6. Efron, N. (1996). Contact lens induced corneal staining. *Optician*, **212**(5558), 18–26.
7. Morris, J. and Stone, J. (1992). The slit lamp biomicroscope in optometric practice – part 1. *Optometry Today*, Sept 7th, 26–28.
8. Morris, J. and Stone, J. (1992). The slit lamp biomicroscope in optometric practice – part 2. *Optometry Today*, Oct 5th, 16–19.
9. Morris, J. and Stone, J. (1992). The slit lamp biomicroscope in optometric practice – part 3. *Optometry Today*, Nov 2nd, 28–30.
10. Veys, J. and Davies, I. (1994). Slit-lamp examination. *Optician*, **208**(5480), 22–27.
11. Woods, R. (1989). Quantitative slit lamp observations in contact lens practice. *J Brit Contact Lens Assoc, Scientific Meetings*, pp. 42–45.
12. Bailey, I., Bullimore, M., Raasch, T. and Taylor, H. (1991). Clinical grading and the effects of scaling. *Invest Ophthalmol Vis Sci*, **32**(2), 422–432.
13. Lloyd, M. (1992). Lies, statistics, and clinical significance. *J Brit Contact Lens Assoc*, **15**(2), 67–70.
14. Mandell, R. (1987). Slit lamp classification system. *J Am Optom Assoc*, **58**(3), 198–201.
15. Jones, L., Veys, J. and Bertrand, P. (1996). Slit lamp biomicroscopy – part 2. *Optician*, **211**(5545), 16–19.
16. Zantos, S. and Cox, I. (1994). Anterior ocular microscopy – part 1: Biomicroscopy. In *Contact Lens Practice*, Vol. 1 (eds Ruben, M. and Guillon, M.), pp. 359–388. Chapman and Hall, London.
17. Efron, N. (1998). Grading scales for contact lens complications. *Ophthal Physiol Opt*, **18**(2), 182–186.
18. Terry, R., Sweeney, D., Wong, R. and Papas, E. (1995). Variability of clinical investigators in contact lens research. *Optom Vis Sci*, **72**(12s), 16.

19. Chong, T., Simpson, TL., Pritchard, N. *et al.* (1996). Repeatability of discrete and continuous clinical grading scales. *Optom Vis Sci,* **73**(12s), 232.

20. Henson, D. (1996). Tonometry. In *Optometric Instrumentation,* Vol. 1 (ed. Henson, D.), pp. 47–79. Butterworth-Heinemann, London.

21. Mishima, S. and Hedbys, B. (1968). Measurement of corneal thickness with the Haag–Streit pachometer. *Arch Ophthalmol,* **80**, 710–713.

22. Mandell, R. and Polse, K. (1969). Keratoconus: spatial variation of corneal thickness is a diagnostic test. *Arch Ophthalmol,* **82**, 182–188.

23. Barrett, B. and McGraw, P. (1998). Clinical assessment of anterior chamber depth. *Ophthal Physiol Opt,* **18**(Suppl 2), s32–s39.

24. van Herrick, W., Shaffer, R. and Schwartz, A. (1969). Estimation of width of angle of anterior chamber. *Am J Ophthalmol,* **68**(4), 626–629.

25. Smith, R. (1979). A new method of estimating the depth of the anterior chamber. *Br J Ophthalmol,* **63**, 215–220.

26. Cockburn, D. (1981). Indications for gonioscopy and assessment of gonioscopic signs in optometric practice. *Am J Optom Physiol Opt,* **58**(9), 706–717.

27. Eperjesi, F. and Barnard, S. (1997). Gonioscopic evaluation of the anterior chamber. *Optician,* **213**(5596), 33–39.

28. Prokopich, C. and Flanagan, J. (1996). Gonioscopy: evaluation of the anterior chamber angle. Part I. *Ophthal Physiol Opt,* **16**(Suppl 2), s39–s42.

29. Prokopich, C. and Flanagan, J. (1997). Gonioscopy: evaluation of the anterior chamber angle. Part II. *Ophthal Physiol Opt,* **17**(S1), s9–s13.

30. Phelps Brown, N. (1995). The Lens. In *Atlas of Clinical Ophthalmology,* Vol. 1 (eds Spalton, D., Hitchings, R. and Hunter, P.), pp. 11.1–11.26. Gower Medical Publishing, London.

31. Meyler, J. (1990). Vitreous disorders in optometric practice: Part 1. *Optician,* **199**(5250), 19–24.

32. Meyler, J. (1990). Vitreous disorders in optometric practice: Part 2. *Optician,* **199**(5252), 19–26.

33. Alexander, K. (1995). Ocular Disease: The Vitreous. In *The Lippincott Manual of Primary Eye Care,* Vol. 1 (ed. Alexander, K.), pp. 126 – 129. JB Lippincott Company, Philadelphia.

34. MacLeod, D. (1995). Vitreous and vitreo-retinal disorders. In *Atlas of Clinical Ophthalmology,* Vol. 1 (eds Spalton, D., Hitchings, R. and Hunter, P.), pp. 12.1–12.24. Gower Medical Publishing, London.

35. Austen, D. (1993). Binocular indirect ophthalmoscopy. *Optometry Today,* March 10, 13–19.

36. Cavallerano, A., Gutner, R. and Garston, M. (1986). Indirect biomicroscopy techniques. *J Am Optom Assoc*, **57**(10), 755–758.

37. Flanagan, J. and Prokopich, C. (1995). Indirect fundus biomicroscopy. *Ophthal Physiol Opt*, **15**(Suppl 2), s38–s41.

38. Johnston, R. (1995). Slit lamp direct ophthalmoscopy. In *Retina, Vitreous and Choroid. Clinical Procedures*, Vol. 1 (ed. Johnston, R.), pp. 89–99. Butterworth-Heinemann, Newton, MA.

39. Barker, F. (1987). Vitreoretinal biomicroscopy: a comparison of techniques. *J Am Optom Assoc*, **58**(12) 985–992.

40. Johnston, R. (1995). Slit lamp ophthalmoscopy using mirrored lenses. In *Retina, Vitreous and Choroid. Clinical Procedures*, Vol. 1 (ed. Johnston, R.), pp. 69–80. Butterworth-Heinemann, Newton, MA.

41. Eperjesi, F. (1997). Slit lamp ophthalmoscopy using mirrored lenses. *Optician*, **213**(5605), 30–32.

42. Bowen, K. (1993). Slit lamp photography. *Spectrum*, **8**(7), 27–33.

43. Cox, I. and Fonn, D. (1991). Interference filters to eliminate the surface reflex and improve contrast during fluorescein photography. *ICLC*, **18**(9/10), 178–181.

44. Lowe, R. (1991). Clinical slit lamp photography – an update. *Clin Exp Optom*, **74**(4), 125–129.

45. Phelps-Brown, N. (1989). Mini pathology of the eye. *Optician*, **197**(5200), 22–29.

46. Phelps-Brown, N. (1991). Ocular photography. *Optician*, **202**(5322), 16–26.

47. Long, W. (1984). *Ocular Photography*. Professional Press Inc, Chicago.

48. Hammack, G. (1995). Updated video equipment recommendations for slit-lamp videography for 1995. *ICLC*, **22**(3/4), 54–61.

49. Cox, I. (1995). Digital imaging in the contact lens practice. *ICLC*, **22**(3/4), 62–66.

50. Krasnow, D. (1997). Set up your slit lamp for video and digital capture. *Rev Optom*, Jan 15th, 47–52.

51. Meyler, J. and Burnett-Hodd, N. (1998). The use of digital image capture in contact lens practice. *Contact Lens Anterior Eye*, **21**(Suppl), s3–s11.

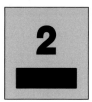

2

Contact lens complications

Lids

Blepharitis

- **Prevalence:** True level unknown, but common (2–5% of all patients). Not contact lens related but likely to impact on contact lens wear.

- **Illumination:** Diffuse illumination.

- **Aetiology:** Two basic types. Seborrheic (oily) and squamous (chronic inflammation or acute infection of the lid margins). Staphylococcal organisms are implicated. Often occurs in patients with acne rosacea and atopy.

- **Symptoms:** Burning, itching and dry, gritty eyes.

- **Signs:** Rosettes – hard, crusting scales on the anterior lid margin at the base of the lashes.
Telangiectasis – dilated blood vessels on lid margin.
Lid margin erythema and oedema.
Tylosis (notching and thickening of the lid margin).
Madarosis (loss of lashes) and/or poliosis (white lashes).
Trichiasis (misdirected lashes).

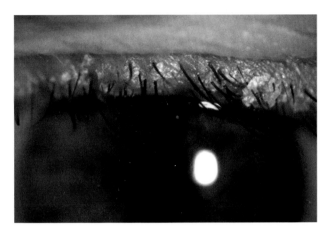

Figure 2.1 Chronic blepharitis. Note the scaly lashes and indurated, thickened lid margin.

Hordeolum — due to acute staphylococcal infections.

Kerato-conjunctivitis sicca (KCS) — present in 50% of patients.

Punctate epithelial keratopathy — in the inferior one-third of the cornea.

Peripheral corneal infiltrates at the 2, 4, 8 and 10 o'clock positions due to hypersensitivity reaction to staphylococcal antigens.

- **Management:** Explain chronicity to patient. Initially warm compresses, lid scrubs (commercial or 'home-made') and artificial lubricants will help. In severe cases oral oxytetracycline/erythromycin (250 mg 4× daily) for 6 weeks in conjunction with either topical fusidic acid gel (fucithalmic) or bacitracin ointment 4× daily for 2 weeks will be required.

- **Prognosis:** Poor. Chronic condition. Patients may continue lens wear once the condition is under control, but cessation of the procedures detailed above will result in a return of the signs and symptoms and invariably contact lens complications and eventual intolerance.

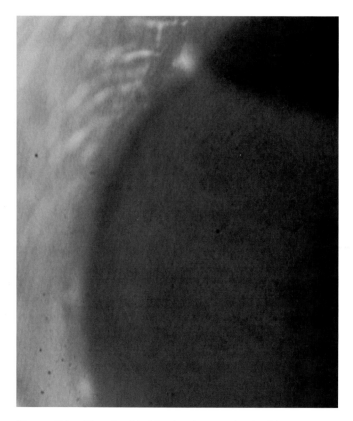

Figure 2.2 Marginal infiltrates in a patient with staphylococcal blepharitis.

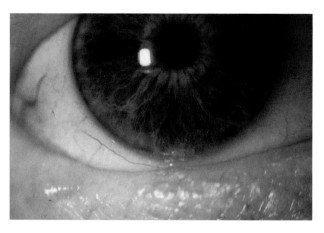

Figure 2.3 Chronic blepharitis changes showing lid margin oedema, tylosis and madarosis.

● References:

1. Dougherty, J., McCulley, J., Silvany, R. and Meyer, D. (1991). The role of tetracycline in chronic blepharitis. *Invest Ophthalmol Vis Sci*, **32**, 2970–2975.
2. Everett, S., Karenchak, L., Kowalski, R. and Roat, M. (1993). Which are the best first-line antibiotics for treating conjunctivitis and blepharitis? *Invest Ophthalmol Vis Sci*, **34** (ARVO Suppl), 851.
3. Fisch, B. (1991). Clinical management of eyelid disease. *Contact Lens Spectrum*, **2**, 40–50.
4. Jones, L. and Jones, D. (1995). Blepharitis. *Optician*, **210** (5522), 32–34.
5. Seal, D., Ficker, L., Ramakrishnan, M. and Wright, P. (1990). Role of staphylococcal toxin production in blepharitis. *Ophthalmol*, **97**, 1684–1688.
6. Seal, D., Wright, P., Ficker, L. *et al.* (1995). Placebo controlled trial of fusidic acid gel and oxytetracycline for recurrent blepharitis and rosacea. *Br J Ophthalmol*, **79**, 42–45.
7. Smith, R. and Flowers, C. (1995). Chronic blepharitis: a review. *CLAO J*, **21**(3), 200–207.

Meibomian gland dysfunction (MGD)

- **Prevalence:** 20–40% of patients. Not directly due to lens wear, but certainly can impact on it. Increases with increasing age, contact lens wear, blepharitis and rosacea.

- **Illumination:** Diffuse illumination.

- **Aetiology:** Obstruction of the gland orifices by desquamated epithelial cells. MGD is a progressive inflammatory process, probably due to the retention of meibum within the glands.

- **Symptoms:** Dry eyes and contact lens intolerance. Possibly some mild pain due to the development of recurrent corneal erosions, secondary to MGD.

- **Signs:** Absent or cloudy meibomian gland secretion upon gland expression. Thickened lid margins, foamy discharge in the tear film and dry eye complications.

- **Management:** The chronicity of the problem must be explained to the patient. In the first instance warm compresses and lid scrubs twice daily and forced expression of the meibomian glands will assist in most cases. In severe cases oral tetracycline 250 mg twice daily for 12 weeks may be required. This will treat both the meibomian gland dysfunction and any associated secondary corneal erosions.

- **Prognosis:** Variable. Dependent upon patients ability to adhere to lid-hygiene regime.

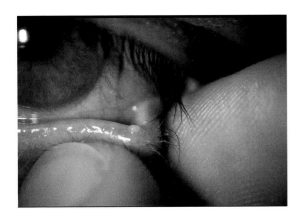

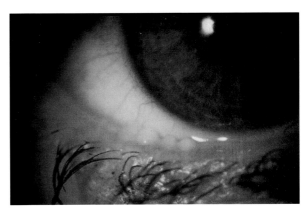

Figure 2.4 Meibomian gland dysfunction showing the technique required to elicit material from blocked glands.

Figure 2.5 Toothpaste-like residue expelled from blocked meibomian glands.

● References:

1. Caroline, P. and Kame, R. (1994). Meibomian gland dysfunction. In *Anterior Segment Complications of Contact Lens Wear*, Vol. 1 (ed. Silbert, J.), pp. 179–192. Churchill Livingstone Inc, New York.
2. Driver, P. and Lemp, M. (1996). Meibomian gland dysfunction. *Surv Ophthalmol*, **40**(5), 343–367.
3. Efron, N. (1998). Contact lens-associated meibomian gland dysfunction. *Optician*, **215**(5641), 36–41.
4. Hom, M., Martinson, J., Knapp, L. and Paugh, J. (1990). Prevalence of meibomian gland dysfunction. *Optom Vis Sci*, **67**(9), 710–712.
5. Hope-Ross, M., Chell, P., Kervick, G. and McDonnell, P. (1994). Recurrent corneal erosion: Clinical features. *Eye*, **8**, 373–377.
6. Hope-Ross, M., Chell, P., Kervick, G., McDonnell, P. and Jones, H. (1994). Oral tetracycline in the treatment of recurrent corneal erosions. *Eye*, **8**, 384–388.
7. Korb, D. and Henriquez, A. (1980). Meibomian gland dysfunction and contact lens intolerance. *J Am Optom Assoc*, **51**(3), 243–251.
8. Ong, B. (1996). Clinical diagnosis and management of meibomian gland dysfunction. *Spectrum*, **6**, 31–36.
9. Paugh, J., Knapp, L., Martinson, J. and Hom, M. (1990). Meibomian therapy in problematic contact lens wear. *Optom Vis Sci*, **67**(11), 803–806.

Contact lens associated papillary conjunctivitis (CLAPC)

- **Prevalence:** Reduced since the introduction of planned replacement lenses. Approximately 5% of soft lens wearers; 2% of rigid lens wearers. More common with extended-wear soft lenses and non-frequent replacement.

- **Illumination:** Diffuse illumination.

- **Aetiology:** Conjunctival inflammatory condition associated with contact lenses, ocular prostheses and post-operative sutures.
  Multifactorial aetiology, probably consisting of a combination of mechanical trauma and immunologically mediated process. Frequently associated with atopy.

- **Symptoms:** Increased lens awareness, foreign body sensation, ocular itching and reduced wear time.

- **Signs:** Large papillary excrescences (>0.3 mm) on the upper tarsal conjunctiva, mucous discharge, tarsal hyperaemia, excessive lens movement and a poorly wetting lens surface. Histologically the conjunctiva thickens and the conjunctival epithelium demonstrates an increase in mast cells, eosinophils, basophils, neutrophils and lymphocytes.

- **Management:** Improve lens hygiene through:
  - daily surfactant cleaning;
  - regular enzymatic cleaning;
  - changing to planned replacement lenses, particularly one-day disposable lenses;
  - changing to fluoropolymer rigid gas-permeable lenses.

  Reduce mechanical influence through:
  - reducing the edge clearance of rigid lenses;
  - reducing the edge thickness of the lens;
  - ceasing lens wear.

Pharmaceutical treatment through the use of:
- topical mast cell stabilizers;
- topical steroids.

● **Prognosis:** Variable. The development of one-day disposable lenses has significantly improved the chances of retaining patients in lenses during the active phase of the disease. Patients who are highly reliant on lenses (such as keratoconics) may require pharmaceutical management during the active stage.

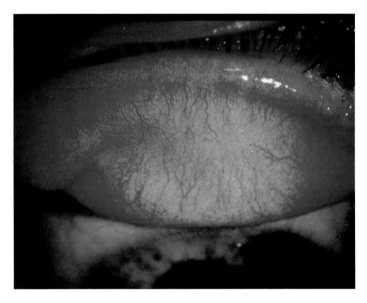

Figure 2.6 A markedly hyperaemic lid in an early case of CLAPC. Note how almost no papillae are visible. (Picture courtesy of Ian Cox.)

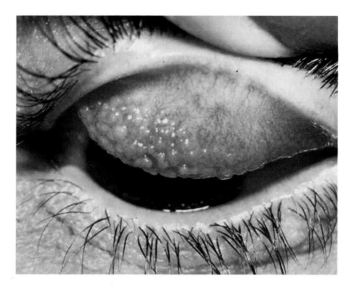

Figure 2.7 Advanced CLAPC. (Picture courtesy of Charles Slonim.)

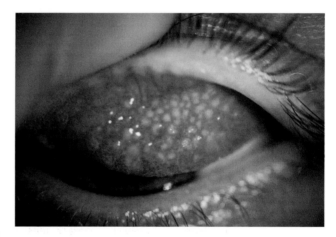

Figure 2.8 Resolving CLAPC in a rigid lens wearer. Note how the apices of the papillae are scarred.

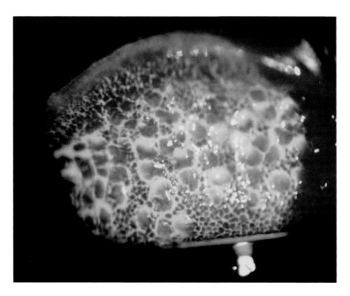

Figure 2.9 The use of fluorescein to reveal papillae height in an active case of CLAPC.

● **References:**

1. Allansmith, M., Korb, D., Greiner, J. *et al.* (1977). Giant papillary conjunctivitis in contact lens wearers. *Am J Ophthalmol*, **83**(5), 697–708.
2. Ballow, M., Donshik, P., Rapacz, P. *et al.* (1989). Immune responses in monkeys to lenses from patients with contact lens induced giant papillary conjunctivitis. *CLAO J*, **15**(1), 64–70.
3. Benjamin, W. (1992). Eyelid travel and the mechanical origin of CL-induced papillary hypertrophy. *ICLC*, **19**(5/6), 143–144.
4. Dart, J. (1986). Contact lens associated giant papillary conjunctivitis. *Contax*, Nov, 6–22.
5. Efron, N. (1997). Contact lens induced papillary conjunctivitis. *Optician*, **213**(5583), 20–27.
6. Jurkus, J. (1994). Contact lens-induced giant papillary conjunctivitis. In *Anterior Segment Complications of Contact Lens Wear*, Vol. 1 (ed. Silbert, J.), pp. 163–177 Churchill Livingstone Inc, New York.
7. Lustine, T., Bouchard, C. and Cavanagh, H. (1991). Continued contact lens wear in patients with giant papillary conjunctivitis. *CLAO J*, **17**(2), 104–107.

Bulbar conjunctiva

Pingueculae

- **Prevalence:** Unknown. Increases with age. Not contact lens related but may impact on contact lens wear.

- **Illumination:** Diffuse illumination.

- **Aetiology:** Degenerative collagen bundles, possibly associated with excessive exposure to dry, windy climates and UV radiation.

- **Symptoms:** Typically none, occasionally mild dryness. Rarely become inflamed (pingueculitis).

- **Signs:** Raised, yellowish nodule on the conjunctiva, usually in a nasal location.

- **Management:** Avoid mechanical trauma through lens striking the raised area. Ocular lubricants are occasionally useful. UV blocking sunglasses may prevent deterioration.

- **Prognosis:** Excellent. Does not interfere with lens wear.

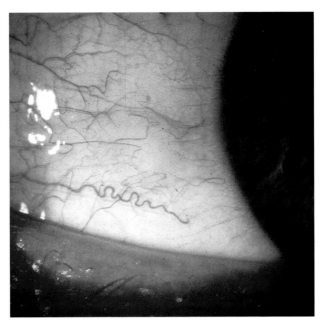

Figure 2.10 Minor pingueculae in a contact lens wearer.

● **References:**

1. Jaros, P. and DeLuise, V. (1988). Pingueculae and pterygia. *Surv Ophthalmol*, **33**, 41–49.
2. Prediger, J. and Edmondson, L. (1993). Management of contact lens patients with pingueculae or pterygia. *Optom Vis Sci*, **70**(1), 9–14.

Pterygium

- **Prevalence:** 2% of all patients. Not contact lens related but may impact on contact lens wear.

- **Illumination:** Diffuse illumination.

- **Aetiology:** Degenerative collagen bundles within the bulbar conjunctiva, possibly associated with excessive exposure to dry climates and UV radiation.

- **Symptoms:** Occasionally dryness. Frequently cosmetic concerns.

- **Signs:** Raised, vascularized nodule on the bulbar conjunctiva, usually in a nasal location, which encroaches on to the cornea and destroys Bowmans membrane.

- **Management:** Avoid mechanical trauma through lens striking the raised area. Minor cases may be managed by occasional use of vaso-constrictors. Surgical removal may be required in severe cases. Ocular lubricants are occasionally useful.

- **Prognosis:** Poor. Rarely interferes with contact lens wear but if the lesion involves the cornea and requires removal then regrowth occurs in up to 40% of cases.

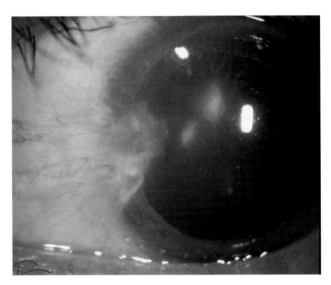

Figure 2.11 Pterygium in a contact lens wearer. Note how the leading edge is overlying the cornea. (Picture courtesy of Anthony Cullen.)

● References:

1. Jaros, P. and DeLuise, V. (1988). Pingueculae and pterygia. *Surv Ophthalmol*, **33**, 41–49.
2. Prediger, J. and Edmondson, L. (1993). Management of contact lens patients with pingueculae or pterygia. *Optom Vis Sci*, **70**(1), 9–14,

Bulbar conjunctival staining

- **Prevalence:**   >95% of contact lens wearers demonstrate some level of bulbar staining, particularly in the nasal quadrant. The degree and presence of staining demonstrates significant variation across time.

- **Illumination:**   Diffuse illumination with fluorescein and barrier filter or rose bengal.

- **Aetiology:**   Probably multifactorial. The degree of staining is increased in dry-eye conditions. Lens-edge staining is due to microtrauma of the conjunctival epithelium through a poor lens fit (rigid or soft) or poor lens edge quality.

- **Symptoms:**   None or occasional dryness.

- **Signs:**   Fluorescein, lissamine green or rose bengal staining of the bulbar conjunctiva.

- **Management:**   None usually required. If due to dry eye – rewetting agents. If due to poor lens fit – modify fit.

- **Prognosis:**   Variable. If due to lens edge, then resolution often occurs by refitting with a different lens type. If due to dry eyes, then total resolution is almost impossible.

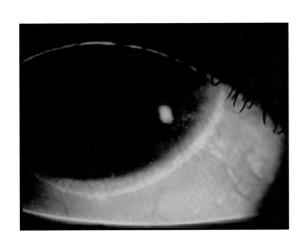

Figure 2.12 Conjunctival staining from soft lens edge.

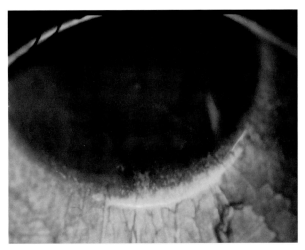

Figure 2.13 Conjunctival staining from rigid lens edge.

● **References:**

1. Lakkis, C. and Brennan, N. (1996). Bulbar conjunctival fluorescein staining in hydrogel contact lens wearers. *CLAO J*, **22**(3), 189–194.
2. Robboy, M. and Cox, I. (1991). Patient factors influencing conjunctival staining with soft contact lens wearers. *Optom Vis Sci*, **68**(12s), 163.
3. Schwallie, J., Long, W. and McKenney, C. (1998). Day to day variations in ocular surface staining of the bulbar conjunctiva. *Optom Vis Sci*, **75**(1), 55–61.
4. Schnider, C. (1994). Rigid gas-permeable extended-wear lenses. In *Anterior Segment Complications of Contact Lens Wear*, Vol. 1 (ed. Silbert, J.), pp. 317–336. Churchill Livingstone Inc, New York.

Bulbar conjunctival hyperaemia

- **Prevalence:** 15–20% of lens wearers, of which 20–35% exhibit clinically significant hyperaemia. Almost 100% of lens wearers will exhibit bulbar hyperaemia at some point in time. Baseline measurements are therefore important.

- **Illumination:** Diffuse illumination.

- **Aetiology:** Major causes include dry eye, hypoxia, a care regimen reaction or poor lens fit. In severe cases non-lens-related causes of red eye (such as keratitis, uveitis and acute glaucoma) should also be considered.

- **Symptoms:** Occasional dryness and reduced lens tolerance.

- **Signs:** Hyperaemia of the bulbar conjunctiva. In rigid lenses the hyperaemia is regional (usually along the horizontal meridian), whereas it is more diffuse in soft lens wearers, suggesting a different aetiology for the two types. It is likely that the hyperaemia with rigid lenses is due to chronic drying whereas that with hydrogel lenses is principally due to a hypoxic cause.

- **Management:** Treat the cause. If severe then cease lens wear. If the situation persists then occasional use of decongestant agents may help cosmesis.

- **Prognosis:** Variable. Certain patients exhibit generally hyperaemic eyes.

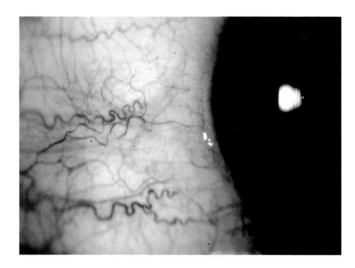

Figure 2.14   Mild bulbar hyperaemia.

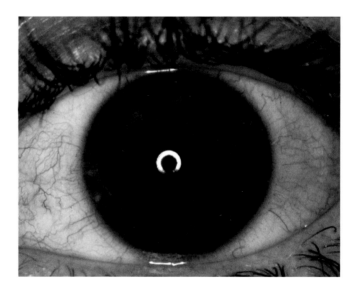

Figure 2.15 Moderate bulbar hyperaemia. (Picture courtesy of Desmond Fonn.)

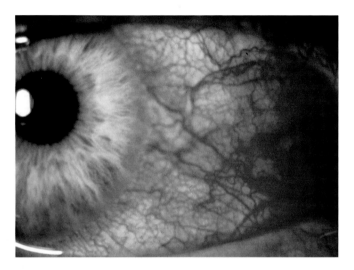

Figure 2.16   Severe bulbar hyperaemia.

- **References:**

1. Efron, N. (1997). Contact lens-induced conjunctival hyperaemia. *Optician*, **213**(5591), 22–27.
2. Guillon, M. and Shah, D. (1996). Objective measurement of contact lens induced conjunctival redness. *Optom Vis Sci*, **73**(9), 595–605.
3. McMonnies, C. and Chapman-Davies, A. (1987). Assessment of conjunctival hyperemia in contact lens wearers. Part I. *Am J Optom Physiol Opt*, **64**(4), 246–250.
4. McMonnies, C. and Chapman-Davis, A. (1987). Assessment of conjunctival hyperemia in contact lens wearers. Part II. *Am J Optom Physiol Opt*, **64**(4), 251–255.
5. Millis, E. (1997). Contact lenses and the red eye. *Contact Lens and Ant Eye*, **20**(Suppl), s5–s10.
6. Munro, F. and Covey, M. (1999). Ocular redness. *Optician*, **217**(5683), 24–34.
7. Pritchard, N., Fonn, D. and Weed, K. (1996). Ocular and subjective responses to frequent replacement of daily wear soft contact lenses. *CLAO J*, **22**(1), 53–59.

Limbal area

Limbal hyperaemia

- **Prevalence:** True degree unknown. Very common in all lens types, particularly soft lenses, with almost 100% of subjects exhibiting some degree of limbal hyperaemia. Clinically significant in 20–40% of subjects. Baseline values are important.

- **Illumination:** Diffuse illumination.

- **Aetiology:** Hypoxia, possibly in combination with mechanical irritation or a tight lens.

- **Symptoms:** Usually none.

- **Signs:** Engorgement of the limbal blood vessels. May be linked to subsequent neovascular changes.

- **Management:** Reduce wear time, increase lens transmissibility and/or optimize lens fit.

- **Prognosis:** Excellent.

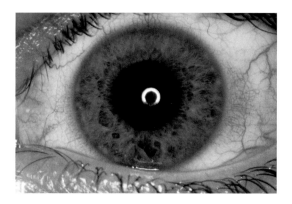

Figure 2.17   Moderate limbal hyperaemia.

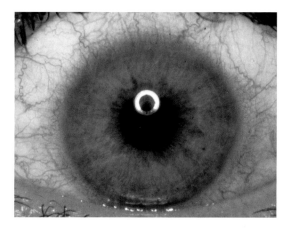

Figure   2.18 Severe   limbal   hyperaemia.
(Picture courtesy of Desmond Fonn.)

● References:

1. McMonnies, C. (1984). Risk factors in the etiology of contact lens induced corneal vascularization. *ICLC*, 11, 286–293.
2. Papas, E., Vajdic, C., Austen, R. and Holden, B. (1997). High oxygen-transmissibility soft contact lenses do not induce limbal hyperaemia. *Curr Eye Res*, **16**(9), 942–948.
3. Pritchard, N., Fonn, D. and Weed, K. (1996). Ocular and subjective responses to frequent replacement of daily wear soft contact lenses. *CLAO J*, **22**(1), 53–59.

Contact lens induced superior limbic keratoconjunctivitis (CL-SLK)

- **Prevalence:** Unknown.

- **Illumination:** Diffuse illumination.

- **Aetiology:** Delayed hypersensitivity reaction to lens deposits and/or care regimen. Typically seen with thiomersolate-preserved care systems, but may be seen with any preserved system. Hypoxia may play a role. Results in bilateral epithelial keratinization and a mild inflammatory response in the area of the superior limbus, under the top lid.

- **Symptoms:** Increased lens awareness, photophobia, burning, itching and reduced wear time.

- **Signs:** Bilateral, superior limbal oedema, a hazy epithelium, superior corneal and conjunctival staining, superior V-shaped fibro-vascular pannus and infiltrates.

- **Management:** In mild cases reduce wearing time only. Severe cases may require a short period without lens wear and non-steroidal anti-inflammatory agents. In all cases prescribe ocular lubricants for interim relief, replace lenses and change to a non-preserved care system or single-use disposable lenses.

- **Prognosis:** Excellent. May take up to a year to resolve completely.

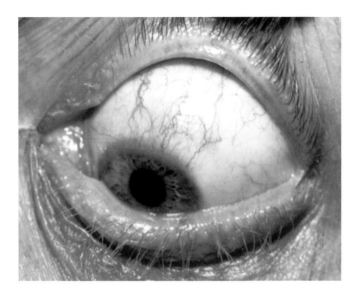

Figure 2.19 Contact lens induced superior limbic keratoconjunctivitis. (Picture courtesy of Anthony Cullen.)

● **References:**

1. Abel, R., Shovlin, J. and DePaolis, M. (1985). A treatise on hydrophilic lens induced superior limbic keratoconjunctivitis. *ICLC*, **12**(2), 116–123.
2. Campbell, R. and Caroline, P. (1996). Contact lens induced superior limbic keratoconjunctivitis. *Spectrum*, **2**, 56.
3. Dart, J. (1986). Thiomersal keratoconjunctivitis. *Contax*, July, 18–22.
4. Efron, N. (1997). Contact lens-induced superior limbic keratoconjunctivitis. *Optician*, **213**(5599), 20–26.
5. Sendele, D., Kenyon, K. and Mobilia, E. (1983). Superior limbic keratoconjunctivits in contact lens wearers. *Ophthalmol*, **90**, 616–622.
6. Stenson, S. (1986). Soft lens-related superior limbic keratoconjunctivitis. *CL Forum*, Dec, 22–24.

Limbal epithelial hypertrophy

- **Prevalence:**   Unknown.

- **Illumination:**   Parallelepiped with fluorescein and barrier filter.

- **Aetiology:**   A tight fitting hydrogel lens acts as a bandage, preventing normal sloughing of the epithelium. Fluorescein pools in the heaped-up areas of the perilimbal cornea.

- **Symptoms:**   None.

- **Signs:**   Fluorescein staining in a band close to the limbus, around most of the corneal periphery.

- **Management:**   Refit with a looser lens if too tight. If lens fit adequate then monitor and refit with different lens design.

- **Prognosis:**   Variable. Certain subjects always show this condition, even on a daily wear basis.

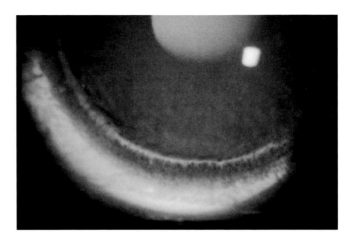

Figure 2.20 Limbal epithelial hypertrophy. (Picture courtesy of Arthur Back.)

● References:

1. Dougal, J. (1992). Abrasions secondary to contact lens wear. In *Complications of Contact Lens Wear*, Vol. 1 (ed. Tomlinson, A.), pp. 123–156 Mosby Year Books, St Louis.
2. Farkas, B. and McGlone, V. (1996). CCR – a hazard of extended wear. *Spectrum*, July, 51.
3. Paragon Optical (1998). Limbal epithelial hypertrophy. *Optician*, **217**(5687), 32.

Staining

Furrow staining

- **Prevalence:**   Unknown. Frequently seen in extended-wear subjects.

- **Illumination:**   Parallelepiped with fluorescein and barrier filter.

- **Aetiology:**   Unknown. May be a variation of limbal epithelial hypertrophy.

- **Symptoms:**   None.

- **Signs:**   Fluorescein pools in groove-like furrows that are perpendicular to the limbus. Most frequently seen inferiorly.

- **Management:**   Monitor limbus for any vessel changes. May be a precursor to oedematous changes. If seen with extended-wear lenses then change to daily wear or consider changing lens design.

- **Prognosis:**   Excellent. Refitting with a different lens design frequently eliminates the problem.

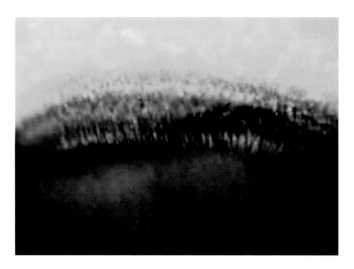

Figure 2.21 Furrow staining. (Picture courtesy of Arthur Back.)

- **References:**

1. Chahine, T. and Weissman, B. (1996). Peripheral corneal furrow staining: a sign to discontinue hydrogel contact lens use. *ICLC*, **23**(6), 229–233.
2. Dougal, J. (1992). Abrasions secondary to contact lens wear. In *Complications of Contact Lens Wear*, Vol. 1 (ed. Tomlinson, A.), pp. 123–156. Mosby Year Books, St Louis.

Superior epithelial arcuate lesions (SEALs)

- **Prevalence:** Published reports indicate that 8% of soft lens wearers exhibit this problem, but newer, more flexible lens types have reduced this figure significantly. The recent introduction of stiffer silicone-hydrogel lenses has resulted in an increased incidence.

- **Illumination:** Parallelepiped or diffuse illumination with fluorescein and barrier filter.

- **Aetiology:** Multifactorial — mechanical, hypoxia and dehydration all implicated. Most likely — mechanical trauma from the inflexible nature of some hydrogel lens designs produces misalignment between lens and ocular surface in the superior corneal periphery due to pressure induced by the top lid. This causes increased mechanical pressure from the lens on the cornea just inside the limbus and produces the characteristic corneal staining.

- **Symptoms:** Often none. Occasionally a foreign body sensation and/or mild irritation upon lens removal.

- **Signs:** Arcuate staining approximately 1 mm from the superior limbus between 10 o'clock and 2 o'clock. The staining runs parallel to the limbus, is 0.1–0.3 mm wide and 2–5 mm in length. Frequently unilateral or asymmetric.

- **Management:** Remove lenses and cease wear for 3–4 days. Resolves in 35% of cases. Fit a thinner, more flexible lens material. Fit a lens with a thinner periphery or fit a flatter back optic radius of the same design. If the problem persists (as in approximately 10% of cases) refit with a rigid lens.

- **Prognosis:** Excellent, although may require refitting with a rigid lens in some cases to eliminate the problem.

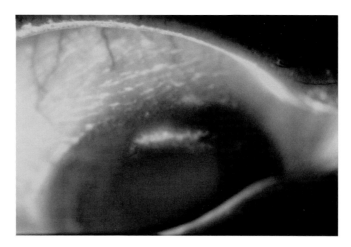

Figure 2.22   Superior epithelial arcuate lesion.

● **References:**

1. Hine, N., Back, A. and Holden, B. (1987). Aetiology of arcuate epithelial lesions induced by hydrogels. *J Brit Contact Lens Assoc Trans Ann Clin Conf*, pp. 48–50.
2. Malinovsky, V., Pole, J., Pence, N. and Howard, D. (1989). Epithelial splits of the superior cornea in hydrogel contact lens patients. *ICLC*, **16**(9/10), 252–254.
3. Young, G. and Mirejovsky, D. (1993). A hypothesis for the aetiology of soft contact lens-induced superior arcuate keratopathy. *ICLC*, **20**(9/10), 177–179.

Inferior arcuate (SMILE) staining

- **Prevalence:** The majority of corneal staining is positioned inferiorly in the cornea.

- **Illumination:** Parallelepiped or diffuse illumination with fluorescein and barrier filter.

- **Aetiology:** Initial lens dehydration, followed by depletion of the post-lens tear film and subsequent staining through epithelial desiccation. Greatest with high water content lenses, thinner lenses, low humidity environments and incomplete blinking.

- **Symptoms:** Occasionally none. Often dryness and reduced wearing time.

- **Signs:** Course inferior punctate staining of an arcuate fashion extending from 4 to 8 o'clock in the lower one-third of the cornea, 3–4 mm in from the limbus.

- **Management:** Minor – no treatment.
  Major – regular use of ocular lubricants, blinking exercises, locally placed humidifiers and switching to either lower water or thicker soft lenses. Persistent cases may require refitting with rigid lenses, although frequently such patients subsequently develop '3&9' staining complications.

- **Prognosis:** Variable. In cases caused by incomplete blinking, complete resolution of the staining is often difficult to achieve.

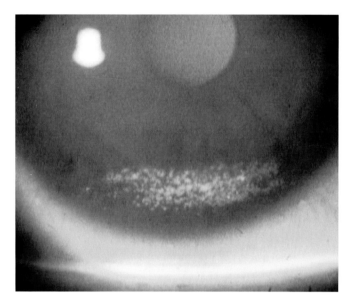

Figure 2.23 Dehydration-induced staining resulting in a typical punctate staining pattern on the lower one-third of the cornea (SMILE).

● **References:**

1. Collins, M., Stahmer, D. and Pearson, G. (1989). Clinical findings associated with incomplete blinking in soft lens wearers. *Clin Exp Optom*, **72**(2), 55–60.
2. Holden, B., Sweeney, D. and Seger, R. (1986). Epithelial erosions caused by thin high water content lenses. *Clin Exp Optom*, **69**(3), 103–107.
3. Jones, L. and Jones, D. (1995). Smile staining and dehydration. *Optician*, **210**(5513), 24–25.
4. Orsborn, G. and Zantos, S. (1988). Corneal desiccation staining with thin high water content contact lenses. *CLAO J*, **14**(2), 81–85.
5. Schwallie, J., McKenney, C., Long, W. and McNeil, A. (1997). Corneal staining patterns in normal non-contact lens wearers. *Optom Vis Sci*, **74**(2), 92–98.
6. Zadnik, K. and Mutti, D. (1985). Inferior arcuate corneal staining in soft contact lens wearers. *ICLC*, **12**(2), 110–114.

Dimple-veil

- **Prevalence:** Unknown. Predominantly rigid lens wearers, rarely soft lens wearers.

- **Illumination:** Parallelepiped with fluorescein and barrier filter and/or indirect retro illumination.

- **Aetiology:** Air bubbles become trapped due to a poor fitting relationship between the cornea and back surface of the lens. Usually observed centrally in steep fitting lenses or peripherally in high riding lenses in cases of high with-the-rule astigmatism.

- **Symptoms:** None.

- **Signs:** Small indentations in the corneal epithelium, resulting in an appearance similar to the surface of a golf ball.

- **Management:** If central dimple-veil, then fit a flatter central back optic radius. If peripheral, reduce the edge clearance, reduce the overall size, control the thickness profile (to reduce the high-riding position) or change to a toric back surface lens in the case of a highly toric cornea.

- **Prognosis:** Excellent. Resolution immediate once fitting relationship between cornea and lens is improved.

- **References:**

1. Jones, L. and Jones, D. (1995). Dimple-veil staining. *Optician*, **210**(5509), 32.
2. Zadnik, K. (1988). A case of dimple veiling/staining. *Contact Lens Forum*, **13**(2), 69.

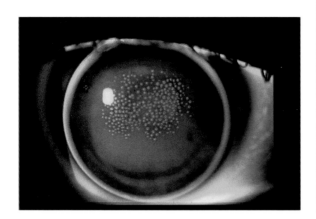

Figure 2.24 Central dimple-veiling in a patient wearing a steep rigid lens. (Picture courtesy of Kathryn Dumbleton.)

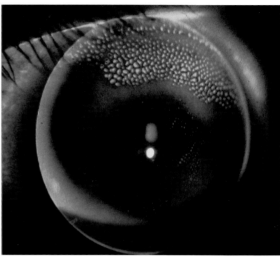

Figure 2.25 Peripheral dimple-veiling in a patient wearing a high-riding rigid lens on a toric cornea.

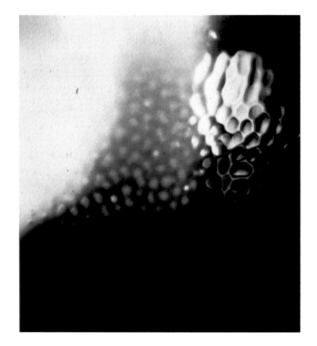

Figure 2.26 Peripheral dimple-veil in a patient following removal of the lens in Figure 2.25. Note the golf ball like appearance of the depressions in the corneal surface.

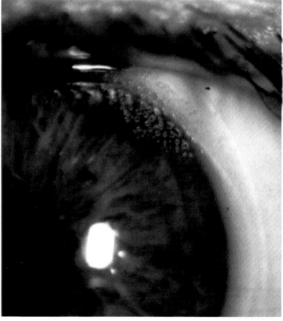

Figure 2.27 Peripheral dimple-veiling in a patient wearing a thick hydrogel lens.

Post-lens debris

- **Prevalence:** Unknown. Significantly higher in extended-wear lenses and appears to increase with the number of nights of extended wear. Also higher in high Dk silicone-hydrogel lenses, possibly due to the high modulus of elasticity.

- **Illumination:** Parallelepiped and/or indirect retro illumination.

- **Aetiology:** Two types are commonly seen. Cellular debris due to epithelial desquamation may become trapped and, following extended wear, balls of mucin may form. Typically these are seen behind a 'stiff' lens following extended wear, particularly with high Dk silicone-hydrogel lenses.

- **Symptoms:** None.

- **Signs:** Mild punctate staining may occur due to the entrapment of cellular debris. Mucin balls appear as spherical, translucent, oily, bubble-like spheres 20–200 μm in size, behind the lens and result in small indentations in the corneal epithelium. The development of such balls under extended wear materials may be due to the collapse of the tear film at night and a subsequent rolling up of the sticky mucin into spheroidal shapes.

- **Management:** Depends upon the severity and cause. The entrapment of cellular debris may result in an acute red eye reaction if not appropriately managed. In such cases changing to daily wear, a looser lens fit or refitting with a reduced stiffness material is indicated. The development of a small number of mucin balls is unlikely to require any management as the condition should not lead to any complications. However, the development of large numbers of mucin balls may indicate an inappropriate lens fit and suitable measures to remedy this should be instituted. Alternatively, the patient could revert to daily wear.

● **Prognosis:**   Variable.

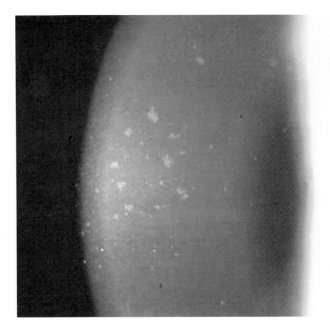

Figure 2.28 Debris behind a thick high water content soft lens. (Picture courtesy of Charles Slonim.)

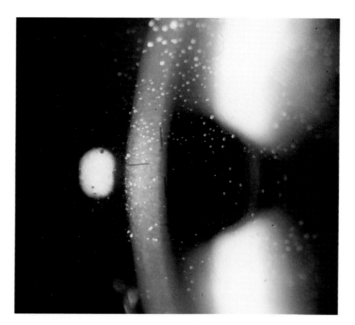

Figure 2.29 Debris behind a high Dk silicone-hydrogel lens. (Picture courtesy of Kathryn Dumbleton.)

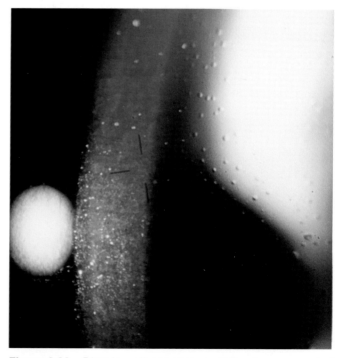

Figure 2.30 Dimple-veil appearance following removal of a high Dk silicone-hydrogel lens that had significant quantities of post-lens debris. Note how the imprints do not display reversed illumination. (Picture courtesy of Kathryn Dumbleton.)

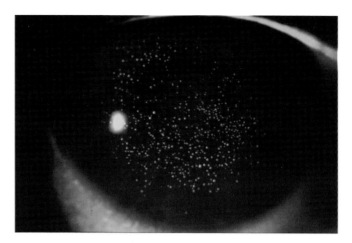

Figure 2.31   Fluorescein imprints following removal of a high Dk silicone-hydrogel lens which exhibited post-lens mucin balls. (Picture courtesy of Kathryn Dumbleton.)

● **References:**

1. Efron, N. (1998). Contact lens-associated blinking disorders. *Optician*, **216**(5667), 18–23.
2. McGrogan, L., Guillon, M. and Dilly, N. (1996). Objective quantification of particle exchange under hydrogel contact lenses. *Optom Vis Sci*, **73**(12s), 100.
3. Pritchard, N. and Fonn, D. (1998). Post-lens tear debris during extended wear of hydrogels. *Can J Optom*, **60**(2), 87–91.
4. Zantos, S. (1984). Ocular complications – corneal infiltrates, debris, and microcysts. *J Am Optom Assoc*, **55**(3), 196–198.

Solution hypersensitivity/toxicity

- **Prevalence:**   1–10% of hydrogel lens wearers.

- **Illumination:**   Parallelepiped or diffuse illumination with fluorescein and barrier filter.

- **Aetiology:**   Toxic changes in the corneal surface due to exposure to elements within a care system. Usually seen in subjects using care systems containing thiomersolate, chlorhexidine or benzalkonium chloride. May also be seen in patients inadvertently inserting lenses directly from hydrogen peroxide without neutralization taking place and in subjects using certain enzyme cleaners.

- **Symptoms:**   Occasionally none. Usually reduced wearing time, dryness and stinging on initial lens insertion.

- **Signs:**   Diffuse punctate staining of the superficial corneal epithelium, generalized conjunctival hyperaemia and occasionally changes to the palpebral conjunctival surface.

- **Management:** Replace lenses, change to a frequent replacement system and/or change to a care system which avoids the toxic product. Soft lens patients could change to a one-day disposable lens and avoid all care system contaminants.

- **Prognosis:**   Excellent.

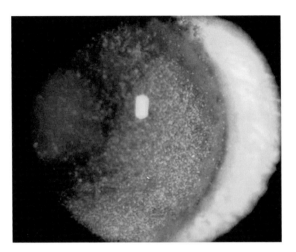

Figure 2.32 Diffuse punctate staining due to a hypersensitivity reaction to a contact lens care system. (Picture courtesy of Ian Cox.)

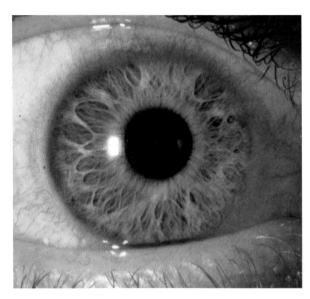

Figure 2.33 Thiomersolate solution reaction. Note the typical circum-limbal hyperaemia.

- **References:**

1. Bennett, E. and Davis, L. (1994). Noninfectious corneal staining. In *Anterior Segment Complications of Contact Lens Wear*, Vol. 1 (ed. Silbert, J.), pp. 41–58. Churchill Livingstone Inc, New York.
2. Caffery, B. and Josephson, J. (1994). Complications of lens care solutions. In *Anterior Segment Complications of Contact Lens Wear*, Vol. 1 (ed. Silbert, J.), pp. 143–161. Churchill Livingstone Inc, New York.
3. Dougal, J. (1992). Abrasions secondary to contact lens wear. In *Complications of Contact Lens Wear*, Vol. 1 (ed. Tomlinson, A.), pp. 123–156. Mosby Year Books, St Louis.

Superficial punctate keratitis (SPK)

- **Prevalence:** Unknown. SPK is a pseudonym for many forms of corneal punctate staining. Some degree of staining may also be seen in non lens wearers.

- **Illumination:** Parallelepiped with fluorescein and barrier filter.

- **Aetiology:** Causes are multitudinal, but central SPK is frequently due to chronic hypoxia, which causes premature desquamation of the stressed epithelial cells.

- **Symptoms:** Occasionally feelings of dryness or 'burning'. Often asymptomatic.

- **Signs:** Pits in the epithelial surface which stain with vital stains, due to damage to the superficial epithelium.

- **Management:** Dependent upon the cause (see management outlines for other forms of corneal staining). If hypoxic in nature, then increase lens transmissibility or change from extended wear to daily wear.

- **Prognosis:** Excellent, if the true cause is isolated and appropriately managed.

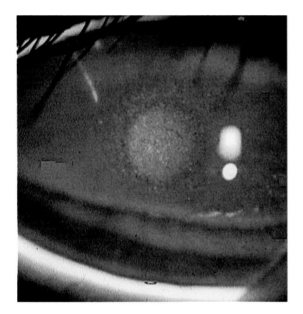

Figure 2.34   Central SPK due to chronic hypoxia in a patient using a PMMA lens.

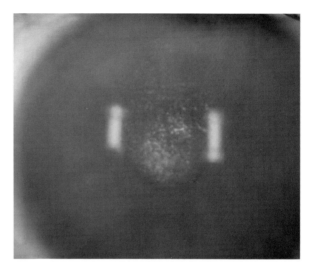

Figure 2.35   Central SPK in a patient wearing a soft lens.

• References:

1. Back, A. (1988). Corneal staining with contact lens wear. *J Brit Contact Lens Assoc Trans Ann Clin Conf*, pp. 16–18.
2. Begley, C., Barr, JT., Edrington, TB. *et al.* (1996). Characteristics of corneal staining in hydrogel contact lens wearers. *Optom Vis Sci*, **73**(3), 193–200.
3. Bennett, E. and Davis, L. (1994). Noninfectious corneal staining. In *Anterior Segment Complications of Contact Lens Wear*, Vol. 1 (ed. Silbert, J.), pp. 41–58. Churchill Livingstone Inc, New York.
4. Brennan, N. and Coles, C. (1998). Adverse effects of corneal hypoxia. *Optician*, **215**(5654), 26–29.
5. Efron, N. (1996). Contact lens induced corneal staining. *Optician*, **212**(5558), 18–26.
6. Schwallie, J., McKenney, C., Long, W. and McNeil, A. (1997). Corneal staining patterns in normal non-contact lens wearers. *Optom Vis Sci*, **74**(2), 92–98

'3&9' staining

- **Prevalence:** Up to 80% of daily-wear rigid lens wearers exhibit some degree. Approximately 15% of subjects demonstrate clinically significant levels.

- **Illumination:** Parallelepiped or diffuse illumination with fluorescein and barrier filter.

- **Aetiology:** Drying of the peripheral cornea in association with an unstable tear film. Causes are multifactorial, including poor peripheral lens fit, inadequate blinking, poor lens wettability and/or abnormal tear composition.

- **Symptoms:** Dry, gritty, irritable eyes and reduced wearing time.

- **Signs:** Conjunctival hyperaemia along the horizontal meridian in conjunction with epithelial punctate staining at the 4 and 8 o'clock positions. Extreme cases may develop a pseudopterygium, vascularized limbal keratitis or dellen.

- **Management:** Fit large rigid lenses with a thin overall thickness profile and low edge clearance, and avoid excessively high or low centring lenses.
  If insignificant corneal astigmatism exists, increase the diameter, reduce the edge clearance, reduce the thickness profile and reduce the edge thickness.
  If significant corneal astigmatism exists, fit a fully back surface toric with a large overall diameter and minimal edge clearance.
  All cases may benefit from blinking exercises and artificial lubricants.
  In severe cases the final resort may be to refit with a soft lens.

- **Prognosis:** In minor cases the prognosis is excellent. In severe cases total elimination of the staining may be impossible (without resorting to a soft lens) and reduction of the staining to a clinically acceptable level may be the best that is possible.

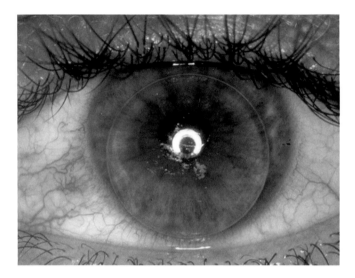

Figure 2.36 3&9 staining, showing the typical horizontal hyperaemia often experienced by sufferers. (Picture courtesy of Desmond Fonn.)

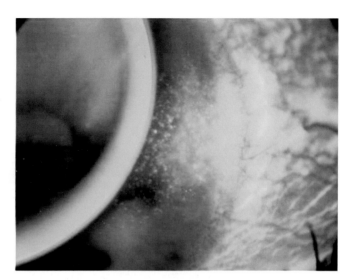

Figure 2.37   Fluorescein uptake in a case of '3&9' staining. (Picture courtesy of Ian Cox.)

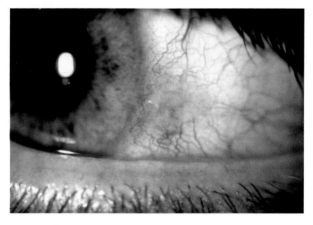

Figure 2.38   Vascularized limbal keratitis in a patient with chronic '3&9' staining

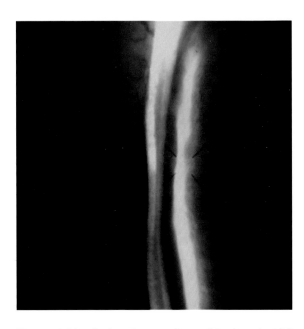

Figure 2.39 Dellen in a patient with chronic 3&9 staining. (Picture courtesy of Kathryn Dumbleton.)

● **References:**

1. Buch, J. (1997). Peripheral corneal staining: a survey of RGP labs. *Spectrum*, May, 31–37.
2. Businger, U., Treiber, A. and Flury, C. (1989). The etiology and management of three and nine o'clock staining. *ICLC*, **16**(5), 136–139.
3. Campbell, R. and Caroline, P. (1995). Dellen formation in RGP contact lens patients. *Spectrum*, **10**(6), 56.
4. Grohe, R. and Lebow, K. (1989). Vascularized limbal keratitis. *ICLC*, **16**(7/8), 197–209.
5. Lebow, K. (1994). Peripheral corneal staining. In *Anterior Segment Complications of Contact Lens Wear*, Vol. 1 (ed. Silbert, J.), pp. 59–90. Churchill Livingstone Inc, New York.
6. Mackie, I. (1971). Localized corneal drying in association with dellen, pterygia and related lesions. *Trans Ophthalmol Soc UK*, 91, 129–145.
7. Schnider, C., Terry, R. and Holden, B. (1996). Effect of patient and lens performance characteristics on peripheral corneal desiccation. *J Am Optom Assoc*, **67**(3), 144–150.
8. Schnider, C., Terry, R. and Holden, B. (1997). Effect of lens design on peripheral corneal desiccation. *J Am Optom Assoc*, **68**(3), 163–170.

Lens binding (RGP adherence)

- **Prevalence:** More prevalent in rigid lens extended wear, in which up to 80% of subjects exhibit binding on eye opening. This is a patient-dependent phenomenon, with approximately 25% of subjects experiencing persistent problems. It can also occur with daily-wear rigid lenses.

- **Illumination:** Diffuse illumination.

- **Aetiology:** Multifactorial:
  - Proposed patient-related factors — high corneal astigmatism, eyelid pressure, peripheral corneal topography, tear film characteristics.
  - Proposed lens-related factors — lens diameter, peripheral curve design, negative pressure, edge clearance, flexibility, lens thickness.

  Most likely explanation is that the lens is pushed down on to the cornea at night by the force of the upper lid, eliminating the post-lens tear film. This leaves only the thin, highly viscous mucus-rich layer, which acts as an adhesive to 'glue' the lens to the cornea.

- **Symptoms:** Frequently none. Occasionally complaints that the lens is difficult to remove and that mild spectacle blur occurs following removal.

- **Signs:** Retro-lens debris behind the mid-peripheral area of the lens and an immobile, decentred lens which leaves an indentation ring when the lens is removed.

- **Management:** To date, published studies indicate that more mobile lenses reduce adherence. To this effect, smaller lenses with increased edge clearance will help to reduce binding. Opinions differ as to whether fitting a slightly steeper or slightly flatter back optic zone radius is preferable. In our opinion, slightly flatter lenses work most often. Additional management strategies include changing to daily wear from extended wear, using frequent replacement rigid lenses or refitting with soft lenses.

- **Prognosis:**   Variable. Inter-subject differences clearly exist and some patients continually have adherence. If the modifications suggested above fail then these subjects must be switched to daily-wear rigid lenses or refitted with soft lenses.

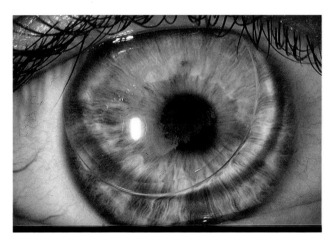

Figure 2.40   Bound rigid lens prior to lens removal. The displaced position of the lens is clearly seen. (Picture courtesy of Cor van Mil.)

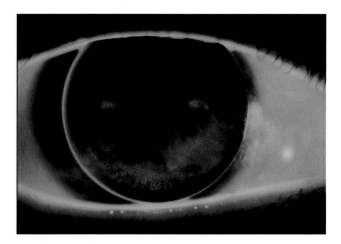

Figure 2.41 Bound rigid lens. The feather-like fluorescein pattern clearly reveals the area of mucin binding. (Picture courtesy of Helen Swarbrick)

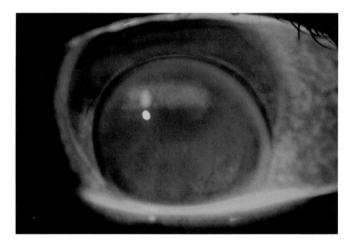

Figure 2.42 Fluorescein appearance on the cornea post lens removal. The area of adhesion is visible at 12 o'clock and the depression in the mucin layer overlying the cornea is visible as a dark line around the edge of the previously bound lens.

- **References:**

1. Eiden, S. and Schnider, C. (1996). Adherence of daily wear RGP contact lenses. *Spectrum*, **2**, 42–46.
2. Kenyon, E., Mandell, R. and Polse, K. (1989). Lens design effects on rigid lens adherence. *J Brit Contact Lens Assoc*, **12**(2), 32–36.
3. Swarbrick, H. and Holden, B. (1991). The clinical correlates of RGP lens adherence. *Optom Vis Sci*, **68**(12s), 105.
4. Swarbrick, H. and Holden, B. (1987). Rigid gas permeable lens binding: significance and contributing factors. *Am J Optom Physiol Opt*, **64**(11), 815–823.
5. Swarbrick, H. and Holden, B. (1989). Rigid gas-permeable lens adherence: a patient-dependent phenomenon. *Optom Vis Sci*, **66**(5), 269–275.
6. Swarbrick, H. and Holden, B. (1996). Ocular characteristics associated with rigid gas permeable lens adherence. *Optom Vis Sci*, **73**(7), 473–481.
7. Woods, C. and Efron, N. (1996). Regular replacement of rigid contact lenses alleviates binding to the cornea. *ICLC*, **23**(1&2), 13–18.

Corneal wrinkling

- **Prevalence:**   Unknown. Most prevalent in thin soft lenses, particularly those of a higher water content.

- **Illumination:**   Diffuse illumination with fluorescein and barrier filter.

- **Aetiology:**   Altered corneal shape due to mechanical pressure from the lens, possibly following dehydration.

- **Symptoms:**   Spectacle blur, which can be significant.

- **Signs:**   Fluorescein pooling in furrows on the corneal surface.

- **Management:**   Refit with flatter lenses and/or thicker lenses which will not dehydrate to the same extent.

- **Prognosis:**   Excellent, if the lenses are suitably refitted.

- **Reference:**

1. Lowe, R. and Brennan, N. (1987). Corneal wrinkling caused by a thin medium water content lens. *ICLC*, **14**, 403–406.

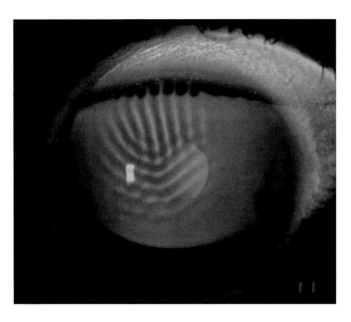

Figure 2.43 Corneal wrinkling following wear of an ultrathin hydrogel lens. (Picture courtesy of Gary Orsborn.)

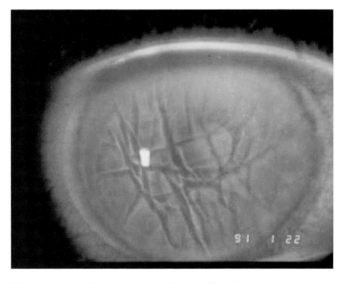

Figure 2.44 Corneal wrinkling following wearing of a pressure patch. (Picture courtesy of Ian Cox.)

Oedema

Epithelial microcysts

- **Prevalence:** Up to 50% of non lens wearers exhibit minimal numbers. Small numbers are observed in 10–20% of daily-wear lens wearers and increased numbers are seen in patients wearing extended-wear lenses or low permeability materials.

- **Illumination:** Marginal retro-illumination.

- **Aetiology:** Hypoxia produces alterations in the mitotic state of the cornea. Pockets of dead cellular matter form adjacent to intra-epithelial sheets at the basement membrane and migrate through the epithelium to the ocular surface.

- **Symptoms:** None.

- **Signs:** 15–50 µm epithelial vesicles are observed in the superficial epithelium some 2–3 months after commencing extended wear. These inclusions display reversed illumination due to their refractive index being higher than the surrounding tissue. If they break through the epithelial surface then the cornea will display a fine punctate staining.

- **Management:** Minor cases (<20 microcysts) require no treatment. If present in greater numbers, then increase the contact lens material transmissibility and/or change from extended wear to daily wear.

- **Prognosis:** Excellent. Initially the number of microcysts increase and then gradually decrease as the mitotic activity within the cornea returns to normal levels. Resolution occurs after 3–4 months.

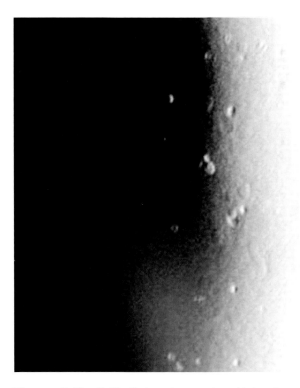

Figure 2.45 Epithelial microcysts. Note how these structures display reversed illumination. (Picture courtesy of Charles Slonim)

● **References:**

1. Efron, N. (1996). Contact lens induced epithelial microcysts. *Optician*, **211**(5549), 24–29.
2. Fonn, D. and Holden, B. (1988). Rigid gas permeable vs hydrogel contact lenses for extended wear. *Am J Optom Physiol Opt*, **65**(7), 536–544.
3. Holden, B. and Sweeney, D. (1991). The significance of the microcyst response: a review. *Optom Vis Sci*, **68**(9), 703–707.
4. Zantos, S. (1983). Cystic formations in the corneal epithelium during extended wear of contact lenses. *ICLC*, **10**(3), 128–146.

Stromal striae

- **Prevalence:** Unknown.

- **Illumination:** Parallelepiped.

- **Aetiology:** Hypoxia results in an accumulation of lactic acid in the cornea, resulting in an osmotic shift within the stroma and subsequent fluid entry into the cornea. It occurs with $>5\%$ corneal oedema and the number of striae proportionally increases with increasing oedema.

- **Symptoms:** None.

- **Signs:** Fine vertically orientated lines in the posterior stroma.

- **Management:** Fit lenses with greater oxygen transmissibility.
  Minimum Dk/t of 24×10^{-9} (cm ml O_2)/(s ml mmHg) for daily wear and 87×10^{-9} (cm ml O_2)/(s ml mmHg) for extended wear.
  Change from extended wear to daily wear.

- **Prognosis:** Excellent.

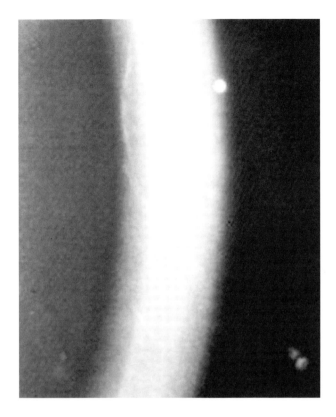

Figure 2.46 Corneal striae. (Picture courtesy of Charles Slonim.)

● **References:**

1. Efron, N. (1996). Contact lens induced corneal oedema. *Optician*, **211**(5540), 18–27.
2. Holden, B., Sweeney, D. and Sanderson, G. (1984). The minimum precorneal oxygen tension to avoid corneal edema. *Invest Ophthalmol Vis Sci*, **25**, 476–480.
3. Holden, B. and Mertz, G. (1984). Critical oxygen levels to avoid corneal edema for daily and extended wear contact lenses. *Invest Ophthalmol Vis Sci*, **25**, 1161–1167.
4. La Hood, D. and Grant, T. (1990). Striae and folds as indicators of corneal edema. *Optom Vis Sci*, **67**(12s), 196.
5. Polse, K. and Mandell, R. (1976). Etiology of corneal striae accompanying hydrogel lens wear. *Invest Ophthalmol Vis Sci*, **15**, 553–556.
6. Sarver, M. (1971). Striate corneal lines among patients wearing hydrophilic contact lenses. *Am J Optom*, **48**, 762–763.

Corneal neovascularization

- **Prevalence:** Approximately 10% of all lens wearers, to some extent. Related to lens transmissibility, with <1% of rigid lens wearers, 5–10% of daily-wear soft lens wearers and 10–20% of extended-wear soft lens wearers exhibiting clinically significant vascularization.

- **Illumination:** Indirect retro illumination.

- **Aetiology:** Hypoxia produces stromal oedema and softening. Subsequent release of vasostimulatory agents results in the ingrowth of vessels into the cornea.

- **Symptoms:** None.

- **Signs:** Bilateral new blood vessels in the cornea. Possibly linked to limbal hyperaemia. Daily wear of hydrogel lenses results in approximately 0.5 mm of vessel penetration and extended wear results in 1.5 mm. More likely to occur superiorly in the cornea due to the reduction in oxygenation under the top lid.

- **Management:** Increase corneal oxygenation by increasing lens transmissibility and/or reducing wearing time.

- **Prognosis:** Excellent. Residual 'ghost' vessels in the cornea may remain many months (or even years) post refitting.

- **References:**

1. Boyce, P. and Carman, S. (1998). A method to quantify vascularization. *ICLC*, **25**, 77–84.
2. Efron, N. (1996). Contact lens induced corneal neovascularisation. *Optician*, **211**(5533), 26–35.
3. McMonnies, C. (1984). Risk factors in the etiology of contact lens induced corneal vascularization. *ICLC*, **11**, 286–293.

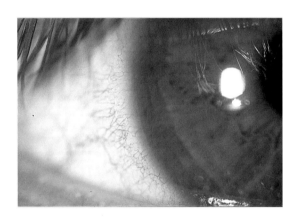

Figure 2.47 Early blood vessel spiking at the limbus. This is frequently indicative of hypoxia and will often result in neovascularization.

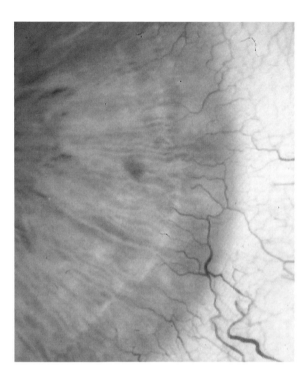

Figure 2.48 New vessel growth in a soft lens wearer. (Picture courtesy of Patrick Caroline.)

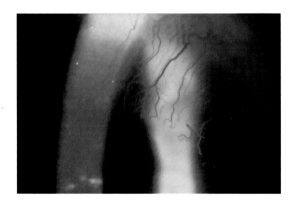

Figure 2.49 Significant new vessel growth under a thick soft lens. (Picture courtesy of Patrick Caroline.)

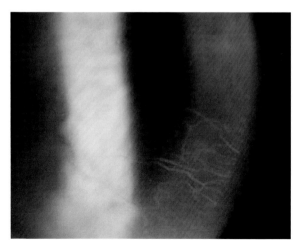

Figure 2.50 Ghost vessels in a patient who suffered from interstitial keratitis. Note the broadness of the new vessels. (Picture courtesy of Anthony Cullen.)

Endothelial polymegethism

- **Prevalence:** Unknown, but endothelial changes are a natural process of ageing. Contact lenses accelerate the process, and the degree of polymegethism is related to the duration of lens wear and degree of hypoxia present.

- **Illumination:** Specular reflection.

- **Aetiology:** Chronic stromal acidosis caused by long-term hypoxia produces structural damage to the endothelial cells, which may result in loss of endothelial pump function.

- **Symptoms:** Usually none, although may be linked to the development of 'corneal exhaustion syndrome'.

- **Signs:** The ratio of the smallest to largest endothelial cells increases from 1:5 to 1:20 and the endothelium is seen to include cells of significantly differing sizes when viewed under specular reflection.

- **Management:** Indicative of long-term hypoxia, therefore refit with high oxygen transmissibility lenses.

- **Prognosis:** Poor. The endothelial appearance never recovers.

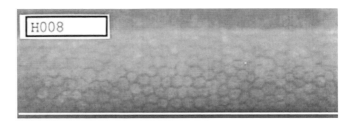

Figure 2.51 Normal endothelial mosaic. (Picture courtesy of Michael Doughty. Reproduced from OPO (1998). 18, 415–422, with permission.)

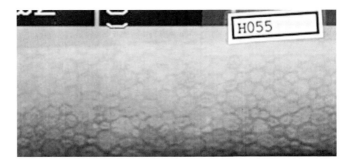

Figure 2.52 Polymegethous endothelial mosaic. (Picture courtesy of Michael Doughty.)

● References:

1. Doughty, M. and Fonn, D. (1993). Pleomorphism and endothelial cell size in normal and polymegethous human corneal endothelium. *ICLC*, **20**(5/6), 116–122.
2. Efron, N. (1996). Contact lens induced endothelial polymegethism. *Optician*, **212**(5575), 20–28.
3. Holden, B., Sweeney, D., Vannas, A., Nilsson, K. and Efron, N. (1985). Effects of long-term extended contact lens wear on the human cornea. *Invest Ophthalmol Vis Sci*, **26**(11), 1489–1501.
4. McMahon, T., Polse, K., McNamara, N. and Viana, M. (1996). Recovery from induced corneal edema and endothelial morphology after long-term contact lens wear. *Optom Vis Sci*, **73**(3), 184–188.
5. MacRae, S., Matsuda, M. and Phillips, D. (1994). The long-term effect of polymethylmethacrylate contact lens wear on the corneal endothelium. *Ophthalmol*, **101**, 365–370.
6. Schoessler, J. (1983). Corneal endothelial polymegethism associated with extended wear. *ICLC*, **10**(3),148–155.

Endothelial blebs

- **Prevalence:** 100% among neophyte contact lens wearers, except those wearing silicone lenses. The level of the response is proportional to the lens transmissibility and reduces in adapted wearers, suggesting an adaptive response.

- **Illumination:** Specular reflection.

- **Aetiology:** Endothelial cell oedema occurs due to a local acidic pH shift (stromal acidosis) due to either an increase in carbonic acid through retardation of carbon dioxide efflux (hypercapnia) or increase of lactic acid due to oxygen deprivation (hypoxia). Bulging of the endothelial cells in the direction of the aqueous produces an optically empty area when the cells are viewed in specular reflection.

- **Symptoms:** Asymptomatic.

- **Signs:** Black, non-reflecting areas within the endothelial mosaic which appear like 'holes' in the endothelium. They appear within 10 minutes of insertion, peak after 20–30 minutes then subside after 2–3 hours.

- **Management:** None required.

- **Prognosis:** Excellent. Blebs disappear within minutes of lens removal.

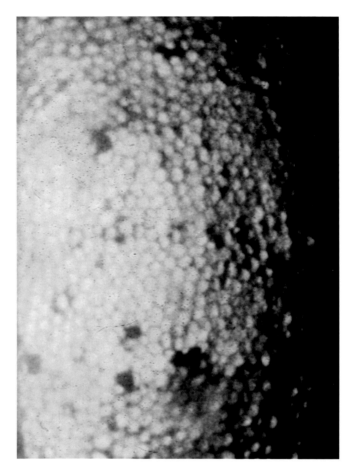

Figure 2.53 Endothelial blebs. (Picture courtesy of Steve Zantos.)

- **References:**

1. Bonnano, J. and Polse, K. (1987). Corneal acidosis during contact lens wear: effects of hypoxia and CO_2. *Invest Ophthalmol Vis Sci*, **28**, 1514–1520.
2. Efron, N. (1996). Contact lens induced endothelial blebs. *Optician*, **212**(5567), 34–37.
3. Zantos, S. and Holden, B. (1977). Transient endothelial changes soon after wearing soft contact lenses. *Am J Optom Physiol Opt*, **54**, 856–858.

Corneal distortion

- **Prevalence:** Up to 30% of long-term PMMA wearers show corneal distortion and spectacle blur is observable in over 90% of PMMA wearers. Often referred to as 'corneal warpage syndrome'.

- **Illumination:** Not visible at the slit lamp. Observed by keratometry, retinoscopy and corneal topography.

- **Aetiology:** Alteration of corneal shape due to chronic hypoxia or poorly fitting lenses. Often seen in patients with significant corneal astigmatism fitted with spherical, low permeability rigid lenses and long-term PMMA wearers.

- **Symptoms:** Spectacle blur upon lens removal.

- **Signs:** Distortion on retinoscopy, distorted keratometry, steepening of the corneal curvature and distorted corneal topography.

- **Management:** Refit with high oxygen transmissibility lenses or improve physical lens fit. Patients are most appropriately managed by immediately refitting with medium to high permeability, well-fitting rigid lenses rather than ceasing lens wear prior to refitting occurring.

- **Prognosis:** Usually good, if diagnosed and appropriately managed at an early stage. Corneal distortion which has not been corrected for many years may not resolve when lens wear is ceased.

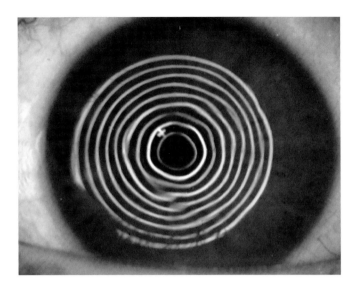

Figure 2.54   Corneal distortion as viewed with a video-keratoscopic device. (Picture courtesy of Patrick Caroline.)

● **References:**

1. Brown, H. (1980). Corneal warpage syndrome – diagnosis and management. *Contact Intraoc Lens Med J*, **6**, 383–385.
2. Hartstein, J. (1965). Corneal warping due to wearing of corneal contact lenses. *Am J Ophthalmol*, *60*, 1103–1104.
3. Levenson, D. and Berry, C. (1983). Findings on follow up of corneal warpage patients. *CLAO J*, **9**, 126–129.
4. Rengstorff, R. (1994). Contact lens-induced corneal distortion. In *Anterior Segment Complications of Contact Lens Wear*, Vol. 1 (ed. Silbert, J.), pp. 351–365. Churchill Livingstone Inc, New York.

Corneal exhaustion syndrome

- **Prevalence:** Unknown, but rare. Only seen in long-term wearers of PMMA or thick, low water content lenses.

- **Illumination:** Not visible at the slit-lamp.

- **Aetiology:** Corneal decompensation due to chronic hypoxia and/or hypercapnia, possibly resulting in endothelial decompensation.

- **Symptoms:** Ocular discomfort, reduced wearing time, excessive corneal oedema and eventually contact lens intolerance, many years after commencing lens wear.

- **Signs:** Endothelial changes, stromal opacification and corneal distortion.

- **Management:** Cease lens wear. Refit with lenses for part-time wear.

- **Prognosis:** Poor.

- **References:**

1. Holden, B. and Sweeney, D. (1988). Corneal exhaustion syndrome (CES) in long-term contact lens wearers: a consequence of contact lens-induced polymegethism? *Am J Optom Physiol Opt*, **65**(12s), 95.
2. Sweeney, D. (1992). Corneal exhaustion syndrome with long-term wear of contact lenses. *Optom Vis Sci*, **69**(8), 601–608.

Corneal hypoesthesia

- **Prevalence:** Unknown.

- **Illumination:** Not visible at the slit lamp. Requires an aesthesiometer.

- **Aetiology:** Corneal sensitivity reduces following wear of lenses that have insufficient oxygen transmissibility, the reduction being directly related to the lens transmissibility. Hypoesthesia is greatest with PMMA lenses.

- **Symptoms:** None.

- **Signs:** Increased corneal touch thresholds.

- **Management:** As a reduction in corneal sensitivity may be indirectly related to epithelial cell repair rate, it is necessary to refit patients exhibiting hypoesthesia with lenses of a higher oxygen transmissibility or to change them from extended wear to daily wear.

- **Prognosis:** Excellent. Recovery rates are related to the degree and length of time under which hypoxia has occurred, but sensitivity will eventually return in all cases, given sufficient time.

- **References:**

1. Bergenske, P. and Polse, K. (1987). The effect of rigid gas permeable lenses on corneal sensitivity. *J Am Optom Assoc*, **58**(3), 212–215.
2. Martin, X. and Safran, A. (1988). Corneal hypoesthesia. *Surv Ophthalmol*, **33**(1), 28–40.
3. Millodot, M. (1974). Effect of soft lenses on corneal sensitivity. *Acta Ophthalmol*, **52**(5), 603–608.
4. Millodot, M. (1984). A review of research on the sensitivity of the cornea. *Ophthal Physiol Opt*, **4**(4), 305–318.

Inflammation (sterile corneal infiltrates) and infection (microbial keratitis)

Inflammation and infection must be differentiated as the aetiology and management of the conditions is very different. Due to the complexities and time involved in obtaining accurate results from cultures, the differential diagnosis is often undertaken using a clinical signs and symptoms 'model', such as that detailed in Table 2.1.

Sterile infiltrates

- **Prevalence:** 1% of non lens wearers, 2–10% of lens wearers. Higher with soft lens wearers (particularly extended wear) and a higher incidence occurs in smokers.

- **Illumination:** Direct focal, parallelepiped. Optic section to assess depth.

- **Aetiology:** An inflammatory response to numerous factors – bacteria, closed-eye environment, tight lens, hypoxia, lens deposits and/or

Table 2.1   Sterile vs. infective keratitis

Sterile keratitis	Infective keratitis
'Presumed' sterile	'Presumed' infective
Inflammatory response	Infective process
Peripheral/mid-peripheral lesion	Paracentral/central lesion
Lesions 1–2 mm	Lesions >1.5 mm
Circular appearance	Irregular appearance
Mild pain	Increasing pain; may be severe
Epithelium – intact or overlying stain	Epithelial staining overlying the infiltrate
Mild epiphora	Intense epiphora
Mild to moderate injection	Moderate to severe injection
Anterior stroma involved only	Anterior to mid-stromal involvement
Mild (if any) corneal suppuration	Severe, progressive corneal suppuration
Minimal anterior chamber reaction	Anterior chamber flare and occasional hypopyon

care systems. Inflammatory cells migrate from limbal blood vessels, forming a white spot in the cornea.

- **Symptoms:** Occasionally none. Foreign body sensation, mild discomfort, photophobia and lacrimation.

- **Signs:** Sub-epithelial focal spots of haziness, normally in the limbal area. Four major types:

  1. Asymptomatic infiltrative keratitis (AIK). Occurs in non lens wearers and wearers of both daily-wear and extended-wear lenses. Focal, often non-staining infiltrates found anywhere in the cornea. Patients are asymptomatic. Causes are unknown, but may be related to low-grade inflammation in response to lens wear or care regimen used.

  2. Infiltrative keratitis (IK). Occurs in non lens wearers and wearers of extended-wear and daily-wear lenses. Focal, usually non-staining limbal infiltrates, generally in the 4 and 8 o'clock positions. Probably related to the release of staphylococcal exotoxins. Requires lid hygiene measures.

  3. Contact lens induced peripheral ulcer (CLPU). Seen in soft lens extended wear only. The infiltrates stain due to loss of full thickness of epithelium and are commonly superiorly positioned under the top lid. Probably due to the presence of staphylococcal toxins or toxins from other gram-positive organisms colonizing the lens. Requires lid hygiene measures and a switch to daily wear.

4. Contact lens induced acute red eye (CLARE). Seen in soft lens extended wear only. The infiltrates rarely stain, rapidly resolve and are usually positioned in all quadrants, close to the limbus. There is an associated marked conjunctival hyperaemia and reoccurrence occurs in up to 50% of patients. Probably due to the presence of gram-negative organisms (e.g. *Pseudomonas* spp.) colonizing the lens or lens case possibly in conjunction with a tight lens. Requires lid hygiene measures, refitting with a looser lens and/or a switch to daily wear.

● **Management:** Dependent upon likely cause. Cease lens wear for 4–21 days, change to daily wear from extended wear, fit planned replacement lenses, change care system, institute lid hygiene measures, loosen lens fit and/or increase oxygen permeability. Some patients may require a short course of topical steroidal treatment to dampen the initial inflammation.

● **Prognosis:** Excellent. Almost all subjects are able to resume lens wear within 2–3 weeks of an episode of inflammation, with no residual complications occurring due to a previous episode. Certain subjects appear prone to the recurrent development of infiltrates and such subjects should be discontinued from extended wear. A scar will remain in subjects who have experienced a CLPU.

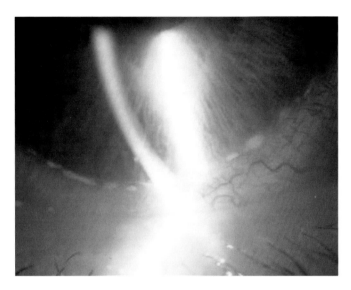

Figure 2.55   Marginal infiltrative keratitis in an extended wear patient. (Picture courtesy of Ian Cox)

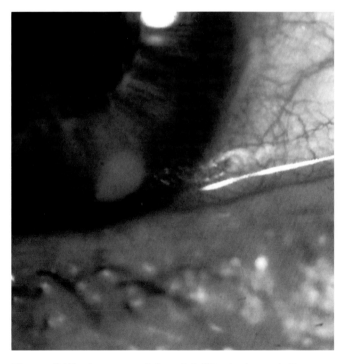

Figure 2.56   Large peripheral infiltrate in a daily wear patient.

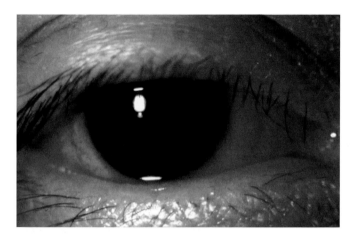

Figure 2.57 CLARE reaction in an extended wear patient.

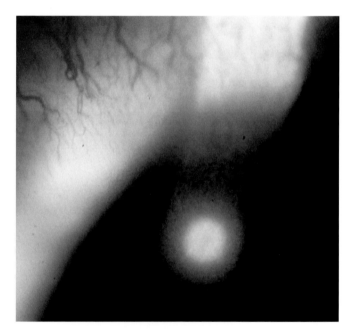

Figure 2.58 CLPU in an extended wear patient. Note how the scar is flat and exhibits no loss of tissue. (Picture courtesy of Karen MacDonald.)

- **References:**

1. Bates, A., Morris, R., Stapleton, F., Minassian, D. and Dart, J. (1989). Sterile corneal infiltrates in contact lens wearers. *Eye*, **3**, 803–810.

2. Cutter, G., Chalmers, R. and Roseman, M. (1996). The clinical presentation, prevalence and risk factors of focal corneal infiltrates in soft contact lens wearers. *CLAO J*, **22**(1), 30–37.

3. Donshik, P. (1998). Peripheral corneal infiltrates and contact lens wear. *CLAO J*, **24**(3), 134–136.

4. Efron, N. (1997). Contact lens-induced sterile infiltrative keratitis. *Optician*, **214**(5608), 16–22.

5. Grant, T., Chong, M., Vajdic, C., Swarbrick, H. *et al.* (1998). Contact lens induced peripheral ulcers during hydrogel contact lens wear. *CLAO J*, **24**(3), 145–151.

6. Holden, B., La Hood, D., Grant, T. *et al.* (1996). Gram negative bacteria can induce contact lens related acute red eye (CLARE) responses. *CLAO J*, **22**(1), 47–52.

7. Silbert, J. (1994). The role of inflammation in contact lens wear. In *Anterior Segment Complications of Contact Lens Wear*, Vol. 1 (ed. Silbert, J.), pp. 123–141. Churchill Livingstone Inc, New York.

8. Stapleton, F., Dart, J. and Minassian, D. (1993). Risk factors with contact lens related suppurative keratitis. *CLAO J*, **19**(4), 204–210.

9. Suchecki, J., Ehlers, W. and Donshik, P. (1996). Peripheral corneal infiltrates associated with contact lens wear. *CLAO J*, **22**(1), 41–46.

10. Willcox, M. *et al.* (1995). Culture negative peripheral ulcers are associated with bacterial contamination of contact lenses. *Invest Ophthalmol Vis Sci*, **36**(4), S152.

11. Willcox, M., Thakur, A. and Holden, B. (1998). Some potential pathogenic traits of gram-negative bacteria isolated during ocular inflammation and infections. *Clin Exp Optom*, **81**(2), 56–62.

Infection (microbial keratitis)

- **Incidence:** 0.04% of daily-wear soft lens wearers and 0.2% of extended-wear soft lens wearers.

- **Illumination:** Direct focal, parallelepiped. Optic section to assess depth.

- **Aetiology:** Bacterial, viral, fungal or amoebic invasion of a compromised cornea. Usually preceded by hypoxia and/or epithelial break. Pathogenic organisms frequently harvested from contaminated lens cases.

- **Symptoms:** Severe pain, photophobia, epiphora and hyperaemia.

- **Signs:** Severe hyperaemia, epithelial staining, area of localized tissue necrosis and frequently an anterior chamber reaction.

- **Management:** Cease lens wear and obtain immediate medical management. Usually involves intensive treatment with fortified antibiotics or fluoroquinolone agents.

- **Prognosis:** Usually good, if referral occurs early in the disease process. Frequently depends upon the causative organism. In all cases a scar will remain. Most patients will be able to resume lens wear.

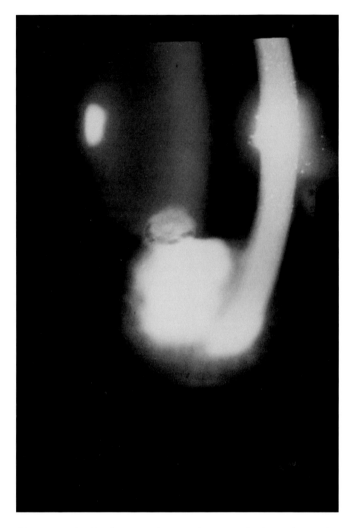

Figure 2.59 Early pseudomonal corneal ulcer. Note the excavated centre to the lesion.

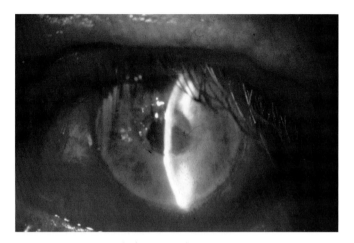

Figure 2.60 Late-stage pseudomonal corneal ulcer. Note the loss of central corneal tissue. (Picture courtesy of Anthony Cullen.)

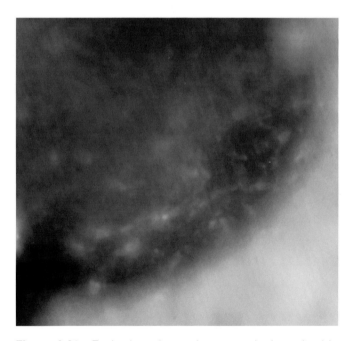

Figure 2.61 Early Acanthamoeba corneal ulcer. In this patient the corneal signs were disproportionate to the intense pain that the patient experienced. (Picture courtesy of Michael DePaolis.)

- **References:**

1. Bennett, H., Hay, J., Kirkness, C., Seal, D. and Devonshire, P. (1998). Antimicrobial management of presumed microbial keratitis: guidelines for treatment of central and peripheral ulcers. *Brit J Ophthalmol*, **82**, 137–145.
2. Cheng, KH., Leung, SL., Hoekman, HW. *et al*. (1999). Incidence of contact lens associated microbial keratitis and its related morbidity. *Lancet*, **354**, 181–185.
3. Dart, J., Stapleton, F. and Minassian, D. (1991). Contact lenses and other risk factors in microbial keratitis. *Lancet*, **338**, Sept, 650–653.
4. Dart, J. (1993). The epidemiology of contact lens related disease in the United Kingdom. *CLAO J*, **19**(4), 241–246.
5. Dart, J. (1997). The inside story: why contact lens cases become contaminated. *Contact Lens & Ant Eye*, **20**(4), 113–118.
6. Efron, N. (1997). Contact lens-induced microbial infiltrative keratitis. *Optician*, **214**(5617), 24–32.
7. Poggio, E. *et al*. (1989). The incidence of ulcerative keratitis among users of daily-wear and extended-wear soft contact lenses. *New Eng J Med*, **321**(12), 779–783.
8. Schein, O., Glynn, R., Poggio, E., Seddon, J. and Kenyon, K. (1989). The relative risk of ulcerative keratitis among users of daily-wear and extended-wear contact lenses. *New Eng J Med*, **321**(12), 773–778.
9. Weissman, B. and Mondino, B. (1994). Ulcerative bacterial keratitis. In *Anterior Segment Complications of Contact Lens Wear*, Vol. 1 (ed. Silbert, J.), pp. 247–269. Churchill Livingstone Inc, New York.

Lens abnormalities

Contact lens deposition

- **Incidence:** Very common. Approximately 80% of hydrogel lenses become significantly deposited over a short time-period. Approximately 30% of all aftercare appointments require remedial action relating to a deposit-related complication.

- **Illumination:** Direct focal, parallelepiped or diffuse.

- **Aetiology:** Patient factors — tear film quality and quantity, hygiene, care regimen. Material factors — water content, surface charge, polymer composition, lens age. Neutral lenses deposit primarily lipid and negatively charged ionic lenses deposit primarily protein.

- **Symptoms:** Reduced vision, comfort and wearing time.

- **Signs:** Variable. Many deposits are not visible. Often lenses exhibit poor wetting. Deposits may be broadly classified into films/coatings and isolated, discrete deposits.

- **Management:** Optimize care system by using surfactant cleaners and/or enzymatic cleaners. Change to deposit-resistant materials or switch to frequent replacement or disposable lenses. This also holds for rigid lenses.

- **Prognosis:** Excellent, if a frequent replacement modality is employed. Some patients will continue to suffer lens deposition regardless of material or care regimen.

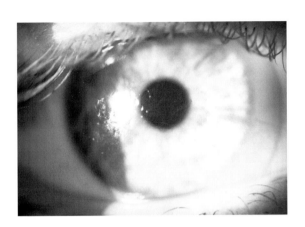

Figure 2.62 Poorly wetting soft lens. This high water content soft lens was 8 months old and had not been cleaned with a surfactant cleaner.

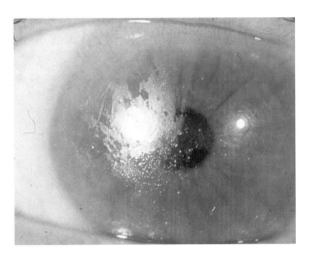

Figure 2.63 Protein film on a soft lens. (Picture courtesy of Charles Slonim.)

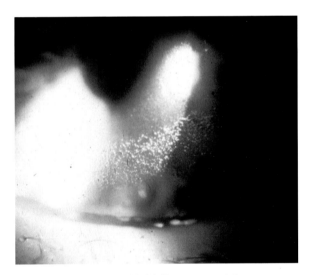

Figure 2.64 Lipid film on a soft lens

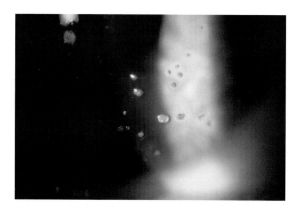

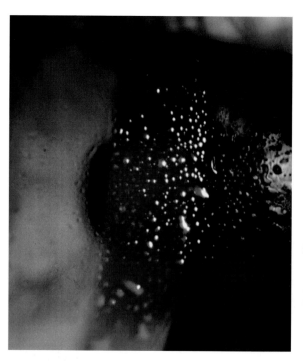

Figure 2.65 Calculi (jelly bumps) on a soft lens. Approximately 90% of this deposit consists of lipoidal material.

Figure 2.66 Greasy, non-wetting rigid lens. Some patients require the use of surfactants containing isopropyl alcohol to prevent the deposition of lipid on the lens material. If seen with new lenses this appearance is often due to poor polishing of the lens during the final manufacture or inadequate removal of pitch.

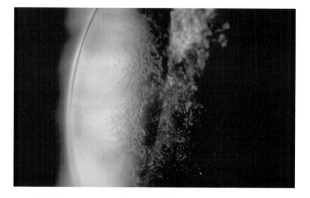

Figure 2.67 Surface plaque on a rigid gas-permeable contact lens. This deposit is thought to consist primarily of lipid and mucin. (Picture courtesy of Patrick Caroline.)

● **References:**

1. Bontempo, A. and Rapp, J. (1994). Lipid deposits on hydrophilic and rigid gas permeable contact lenses. *CLAO J*, **20**(4), 242–245.
2. Hart, D., Tidsale, R. and Sack, R. (1986). Origin and composition of lipid deposits on soft contact lenses. *Ophthalmol*, **93**(4), 495–503.
3. Jones, L. (1993). Contact lens deposits: their causes and control. *Contact Lens J*, **20**(1), 6–13.
4. Jones, L., Franklin, V., Evans, K., Sariri, R. and Tighe, B. (1996). Spoilation and clinical performance of monthly vs. three monthly disposable contact lenses. *Optom Vis Sci*, **73**(1), 16–21.
5. Jones, L., Evans, K., Sariri, R., Franklin, V. and Tighe, B. (1997). Lipid and protein deposition of N-vinyl pyrrolidone containing group II and group IV frequent replacement contact lenses. *CLAO J*, **23**(2), 122–126.
6. Leahy, C., Mandell, R. and Lin, S. (1990). Initial in vivo tear protein deposition on individual hydrogel contact lenses. *Optom Vis Sci*, **67**(7), 504–511.
7. Maissa, C., Franklin, V., Guillon, M. and Tighe, B. (1998). Influence of contact lens material surface characteristics and replacement frequency on protein and lipid deposition. *Optom Vis Sci*, **75**(9), 697–705.
8. McMonnies, C. (1991). Surface deposit theory and practice. *J Brit Contact Lens Assoc*, **14**(4), 179–182.
9. Minarik, L. and Rapp, J. (1989). Protein deposits on individual hydrophilic contact lenses: effects of water and ionicity. *CLAO J*, **15**(3), 185–188.
10. Rapp, J. and Broich, J. (1984). Lipid deposits on worn soft contact lenses. *CLAO J*, **10**(3), 235–239.
11. Sack, R., Jones, B., Antignani, A., Libow, R. and Harvey, H. (1987). Specificity and biological activity of the protein deposited on the hydrogel surface. *Invest Ophthalmol Vis Sci*, **28**(5), 842–849.
12. Tighe, B., Bright, A. and Franklin, V. (1991). Extrinsic factors in soft contact lens spoilation. *J Brit Contact Lens Assoc*, **14**(4), 195–200.
13. Tighe, B. and Franklin, V. (1997). Lens deposition and spoilation. In *The Eye in Contact Lens Wear*, Vol. 1 (ed. Larke, J.), pp. 49–100. Butterworth-Heinemann, Oxford.
14. Tripathi, R., Tripathi, B. and Silverman, R. (1994). Morphology of lens deposits and causative effects. In *Contact Lens Practice*, Vol. 1 (eds Ruben, M. and Guillon, M.), pp. 1099–1117. Chapman and Hall, London.

Damage

- **Incidence:** Unknown. Frequently a higher incidence is found in new wearers or hypermetropes due to inadequate handling technique or difficulties with locating the lens. As a general rule, lens life is related to lens permeability, with higher permeability lenses having a shorter lens life, when used on a daily-wear basis.

- **Illumination:** Diffuse or direct focal, parallelepiped.

- **Aetiology:** Usually due to poor handling or trapping the lens edge in the lens case.

- **Symptoms:** Frequently none. Occasionally minor lens irritation and foreign body sensation, which ceases following lens removal.

- **Signs:** Splits or cracks within the lens or a segment missing from the lens edge. Occasionally the area adjacent to the damage will exhibit corneal staining.

- **Management:** Replace lens and review handling procedures.

- **Prognosis:** Excellent. If damage continually occurs then consider changing to a frequent replacement programme.

- **References:**

1. Dougal, J. (1992). Abrasions secondary to contact lens wear. In *Complications of Contact Lens Wear*, Vol. 1 (ed. Tomlinson, A.), pp. 123–156. Mosby Year Book, St Louis.
2. Jones, L., Woods, C. and Efron, N. (1996). Life expectancy of rigid gas permeable and high water content contact lenses. *CLAO J*, **22**(4), 258–261.

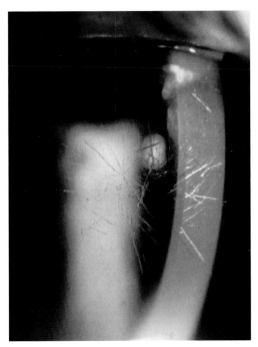

Figure 2.68   Scratched rigid gas-permeable lens.

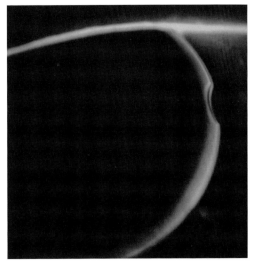

Figure 2.69   PMMA lens with a section broken off the edge. This lens was still being worn by the patient, who was unaware of the broken edge.

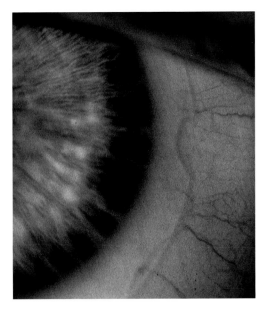

Figure 2.70   Torn soft lens.

Excellent reviews of complications may be found in a number of texts, including those listed below. Interested readers are referred to these and the references included for further detailed information.

1. Anderson, J., Davies, I., Kruse, A. *et al.* (1995). *A Handbook of Contact Lens Management*. Vistakon, Jacksonville.
2. Brennan, N. and Bruce, A. (1995). *A Guide to Clinical Contact Lens Management*. CIBA Vision, Atlanta.
3. Bruce, A. and Brennan, N. (1990). Corneal pathophysiology with contact lens wear. *Surv Ophthalmol*, **35**(1), 25–58.
4 Covey, M. and Munro, F. (1999). Differential diagnosis in contact lens aftercare. *Optician*, **217**(5691), 24–32.
5. Efron, N. (1999). *Contact Lens Complications*. Butterworth-Heinemann, Oxford.
6. Silbert, J. (1994). *Anterior Segment Complications of Contact Lens Wear*. Churchill Livingstone Inc, New York.
7. Stapleton, F. and Dart, J. (1995). Management of contact lens related disease. *Optician*, **210**(5530), 21–26.
8. Tomlinson, A. (1992). *Complications of Contact Lens Wear*. Mosby Year Books, St Louis.

Index